I Choose To Be Happy

Happiness Comes From Within

Marie Elson

Energy Wizard and International Bestselling Author

I Choose To Be Happy

From someone enjoying a long and happy life comes this little book of musings, wisdom, advice, inspiration, spirituality, stories of family togetherness and love and friendship, wellness and healing techniques and therapies, and delicious traditional recipes.

All for the cultivation and achievement of HAPPINESS!

About the Author

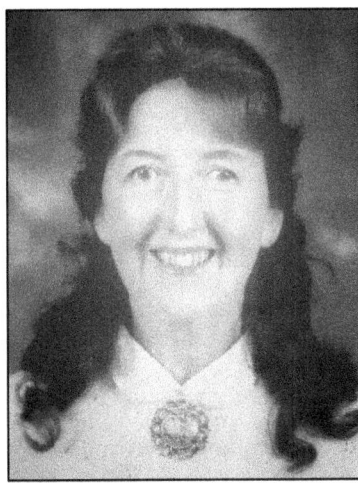

Marie Elson has always lived with inner happiness and appreciation of her remarkable life. For many years Marie has been involved with all areas of inner peace and the advancement of joy, and now wishes for others to be blessed with the knowledge and skills to THINK happy, DO happy, and BE happy. She has offered many years of housesitting in Australia, along with writing, puzzling, and continuing her passion for gardening. She is now indulging in joyous activities while living her dream retirement life beachside in Capel Sound, Victoria.

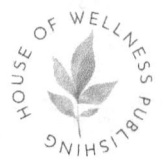

DISCLAIMER

Copyright © 2024 House of Wellness Publishing.

All rights reserved.

No part of this publication may be reproduced, stored in a retrieval system, or transmitted in any form or by any means, electronic, mechanical, photocopying, recording, or otherwise, without the copyright owner's and publisher's prior written permission. Nothing in this book should be considered as medical advice, and readers should consult their own health professionals when making decisions about their own health and medical or therapeutic treatments. Should any reader choose to use the information contained herein, this is their decision, and the author and publishers do not assume any responsibilities under any circumstances.

References:
All website links provided are correct at time of first publication.

Contents

1. An Introduction to Happiness — 6

2. The Happiness Alphabet — 9

3. Healing Myself for Happiness — 66

4. One More Note of Happiness — 84

Quick Finder – Recipes Index — 86

Contributions to Other Publications — 87

Praise for 'I Choose To Be Happy' — 88

Author's Message and Thanks — 89

Publisher's Message (Get in Touch!) — 91

1. An Introduction to Happiness.

I start to dig a hole for my new rose, Angel Face, in our new front garden space. We have not long moved into our new beach villa home and it's time to make it our own. I had dreamed for many years of this very day, to finally be living here beachside at Rosebud. My daughter has just presented me with one of my favourite roses. We have a rose for each family member, and this is hers that she has gifted me herself – Angel Face.

I have so many wonderful memories of summer holidays our family took at Rosebud Beach, after travelling down from the city. When my daughter was a small child, she would run for hours on the vast expanse of beach as the tide went out. Many years of sunsets, fish and chips beach picnics (mainly feeding the seagulls, I feel) and many sea-misty mornings. I'm looking forward to beachside adventures again in our joyous newness.

However, the weather can no longer be trusted, and I am successful at planting Angel Face just as the inclemency arrives, but I carry on for this brings me great happiness. *La pluie* is falling drop after drop and I'm still enjoying this moment, as I always have – being in the outdoors and elements, being present in the garden. It's my lifeline; I come from a very long line of green-thumbs, with cooking, baking and preserving also bringing me just as much happiness and joy. The secret to happiness is to be a happy person from within, no matter the weather.

Happiness is a light and lovely part of life, so why should we learn about it in large and complicated books that can be heavy and difficult to read and comprehend?

This is a small book with a big message.

It is light and airy, easy to understand, not complex, accessing my family traditions, informative, interesting, and easy to follow. This will warm you and provide you with 'you time', patience, and perseverance strategies. But this book is not for those with a lazy attitude – your contribution will be needed to follow along, understand, and accept the applications with diligence. Your time and effort will be required to implement and then create the happiness you desire in your life. Other people will not provide happiness for you, and you cannot wait around for happiness to just arrive, either – you must do it yourself. It's time to change your thought patterns around happiness as not something you 'get' or simply just 'feel', but a state you create to **BE**. To feel happy you need to BE happy first and create happy feelings. Yes, it's work time, time to work on YOU to be happy for yourself.

The secret to happiness is the choice to be a happy person.

In a world of counting money, steps and calories, let's be rebels and count our blessings, our happy moments, our laughter, and our joy. Let *le soleil* come out and flood your days with light.

SUNSHINE CAKE

TAKE: One tablespoon of Trouble

ADD: Two Smiles, and let it bubble

GENTLY ADD:

One cup of Love

One cup of Light

One cup of Loveliness

METHOD: Look in your heart until it shines, and VOILÀ…

* **SUNSHINE CAKE** *

This cake is so easy to make. Your 'cake tin' will always be full, and it will remain perfectly clean, too!

MAY THE SUN ALWAYS SHINE ON YOU!

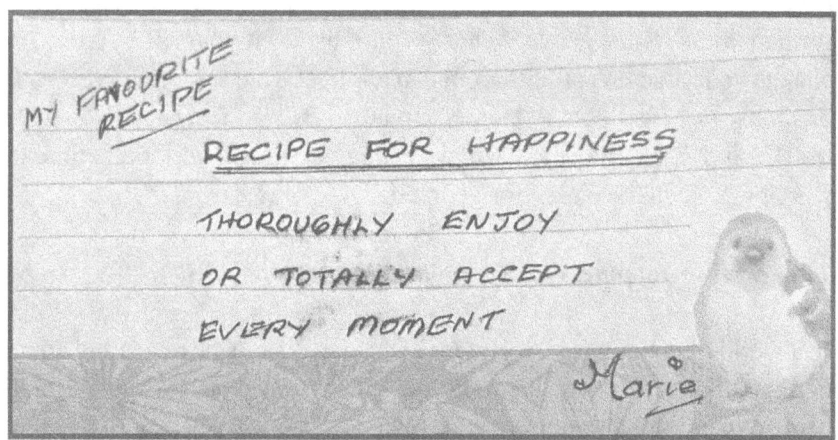

MY FAVOURITE RECIPE

RECIPE FOR HAPPINESS

THOROUGHLY ENJOY OR TOTALLY ACCEPT EVERY MOMENT

Marie

2. The Happiness Alphabet.

If something that you had just finished reading was most interesting and contained 500 pages and thousands of words, you would probably remember many of those words. If you read something containing 100 pages, perhaps you would remember even more of the words. And if you read a one-page article you might even remember most of it.

The memory says: "Fewer words – easy to remember, thank you." When we want to deliver an important message that needs to be remembered, a handful of really relevant and descriptive words is often sufficient (e.g., 'be kind, always and in all ways'). The brain can readily accept a short message and retain it in the memory bank.

In this chapter I have some short-message 'ABCs' for you to consider for creating your happiness. After my short messages I've also included some supplementary 'happiness-promotion material' in the form of a Garden Tip, a Natural Therapy Thought, and a Favourite Recipe (or Favourite Food Thought) for each letter.

I suggest that you learn to apply the little A-Z messages to your day-today life to create the basics of your happiness. And if you also find something useful or enjoyable in the supplementary material, then that will only add to the development of your happy life! You can then encourage and nurture others to be happy, too.

Remember, happiness is something you THINK and DO and BE, and not something that just happens to you, somehow, sometimes.

So, I hope that you will enjoy and find great success within these ABCs for a back-to-basics approach to happiness and wellbeing creation.

A.   'A' IS FOR 'APPRECIATE LIFE'

Appreciate your life and accept everything it presents to you.

There are numerous ups and downs in life and we have to face them, all of them – the good, the bad, the easy, the difficult. When we are feeling 'up' and things are freely flowing, we are happy with life. When the 'downs' arrive, we tend to go down with them and allow unhappiness to creep in. But it does not have to be this way. Understand that you now have something on which to work – accept it, get working, and move on, always remembering that more good times are ahead. Thoroughly enjoy the highs, and learn from the lows.

Three important things to remember:
- Appreciate the positives and learn from the negatives in your life.
- Appreciate that natural, healthy foods are best for you.
- Appreciate that fresh air and sunshine are a MUST.

Garden Tip 'A':
- *African violet.*

This was one of my mother's most favourite plants (all violets, actually –

Mother loved their 'little smiling faces'). The African violet is a very popular houseplant grown for its gorgeous blooms, durability and prowess for sugaring for cake decoration (one of my old favourite hobbies from many years ago now).

Natural Therapy Thought 'A':
- *Homeopathic arnica.*

I worked for a homeopath for many years, Mr Hainsworth Cock, and the knowledge I gained has been life-changing – not only for my own knowledge, but for my family's health too. The Cock family became great family friends, and I am proud to mention them in my publication. Arnica has been a godsend over the years as a part of the 'Homeopathic ABC' (arnica, belladonna, chamomile) protocol for emergency health, and individually for first aid, and bruising and wound care.

Favourite Recipe 'A':
- *Apple and rhubarb crumble.*

My mother and father were prolific gardeners. Flowers and blooms were out front and were Mother's pride and joy, while a market vegetable garden (Dad was an AMAZING vegetable gardener), a mini-orchard and a chicken coop were out the back. They grew two kinds of apples and the most delicious rhubarb.

Enjoy this recipe with grace (we all called Mother 'Amazing Grace'!).

INGREDIENTS
- Tart apples, 3 cups
- Fresh rhubarb, 2 sticks
- Water (for stewing)
- Sugar, *1/2* cup for fruit preparation plus another *1/2* cup for the crumb
- Rolled oats, 2 cups
- Plain flour, 1 cup
- Butter, 60 g

- Maple syrup or honey (for drizzling)
METHOD
- Peel and quarter a tart type of apple, such as Granny Smith (Mother's choice was snow apples) to get three cups in total.
- Peel and dice the sticks of fresh rhubarb.
- Stew the apple and rhubarb together in a saucepan with a little water and a half-cup of sugar, until the fruit is soft. Leave to cool.
- For the crumb, place the rolled oats, plain flour, remaining half-cup of sugar and the butter in a bowl and rub with fingertips until the mixture resembles crumbs.
- Place the stewed fruit in your choice of dessert baking dish and cover with the crumb mix. Squeeze on drizzles of maple syrup or honey.
- Bake for 30 minutes at 180 degrees Celsius or until the top is golden brown.

B.   'B' IS FOR 'BED IS FOR SLEEPING'

Your bedroom is your sleep place.

Make sure you treat your bedroom as your temple for sleep rather than using it as an office or entertainment centre. Most homes have sufficient space in other areas for computers, TVs, etc., which can be enjoyed before bedtime. It is important, especially for light sleepers, to keep reminding the body that the bedroom is a place to relax and sleep. Treat your bed as a friend – visit it regularly. A regular sleeping habit is most important, and it is a good idea to get some quality sleep before midnight.

Three important things to remember:
- Your bedroom is your 'sleep place'.
- Your bedroom is not an entertainment centre.
- Plan to have some sleep before midnight.

Garden Tip 'B':
- *Blooms.*

Grow yourself some flowers, admire their pretty faces, smell them, enjoy them, even plant edible blooms like calendula, nasturtiums, roses, borage; and enjoy them with gratitude and grace. If you can't grow them, buy yourself some. Flowers are the decorations of life. The garlands of nature to enjoy.

The best tip for growing flowers is to choose some that suit your climate, and then water and fertilise them in the appropriate way that they require – don't just go in blindly. Nurture them and they will nurture you in return and adorn you with colour. Choose something aromatic so you can sniff them too.

Natural Therapy Thought 'B':
- *Basket-weaving.*

Would you believe that my father indulged me with basket-weaving? We would purchase cane lengths, soak them in water, and construct the basket bases of varied shapes and sizes. After making the right holes we then placed vertical non-soaked cane in the bases to become the mainframe of the basket, then wove the malleable cane crosswise from the base up to the top to complete the basket. Dad would always finish his baskets off with a decorative filigree rim, which received many comments of praise. We went into basket production pretty much full-time for a few years. Our final products were used as hampers, fishing traps, gift baskets, storage baskets, and even as display containers for dried flower arrangements. I have such fond memories of our pastime together and the very specific skillset we had. Many years later, my husband and I sent our daughter to Rudolph Steiner School, where lots of art and handicrafts were undertaken as part of the curriculum and by participating families, and so our basket-weaving continued. Trust me, and give basket-weaving a go.

Favourite Recipe 'B':
- *Banana bread.*

My sister-in-law was well known for her magnificent banana bread, making it for family and friends for over 60 years. I'm delighted to share her recipe here. And now the cat is out of the bag – the secret to an ever-so-moist banana bread is to use many overripe (even black!) bananas. The cake sticks to the back of your fork – yum!

<u>INGREDIENTS</u>
- Overripe (black and squishy!) bananas, 4
- Eggs, 3
- Butter, 1 cup (melted and cooled)
- Buttermilk, 1 cup
- Self-raising flour, 2 cups
- Cream cheese frosting (optional)

<u>METHOD</u>
- Thoroughly mash the bananas.
- Use a mixer to beat the banana mash, eggs, butter liquid and buttermilk until smooth. Fold in the self-raising flour until combined.
- Place in a greased and lined loaf tin and bake at 160 degrees Celsius for 40 minutes.
- Cool the loaf fully. Ice with cream cheese frosting, if desired (beat your chosen quantity of cream cheese with icing sugar – AKA powdered sugar – and vanilla essence, to desired taste and consistency).

C.   'C' IS FOR 'CARE ABOUT EVERYTHING'

Caring leads to sharing, and both lead to happiness.

It is really important to care about life in general. Care about your family, your friends, and your fellow human beings, as well as about your environment and all it involves, including yourself.

Three important things to remember:
- Care about and respect yourself, your family, your friends and others.
- Take good care of your home and the environment.
- Care enough to reach out and help others when they need it.

Garden Tip 'C':
- *Calendulas.*

Calendulas are one of my daughter's absolute favourites to grow. Not only do they present wonderfully colourful flower faces and make colourful garden beds, but they are also an excellent companion plant in gardening to deter pestilent insects. They are a great medicinal herb and the petals make a wonderful tea, useful as a liver tonic, a calmative, a hair and skin rejuvenator, and a sleep tonic. I think calendulas are a must-have in your garden or patio pots.

Natural Therapy Thought 'C':
- *CURIOSITY!*

By harbouring an intense sense of wonder and curiosity you will find enrichment and joy at every corner. I wonder, what will tomorrow bring you? Do you think you don't care, or are 'bored'? (I don't believe in that word, by the way!)

Here are some tips on how to be more curious.
- Determine what intrinsically motivates you.
- Ask better questions in conversations. Be willing to ask dumb questions, too!
- Challenge your assumptions, thoughts, and preconceived ideas.
- Make an effort to learn daily. Read more and read widely, and follow your interests.
- SHARE. For example, share something you have learned from reading here – has something motivated you to action a piece of my information? Has something piqued your interest and you want to investigate it further on your own?

There are some surprising benefits of being a curious person. Curiosity helps us survive. The urge to explore and seek novelty helps us remain vigilant and offers mental stability. Curious people are happier – research has shown curiosity to be associated with higher levels of positive feelings. Curiosity boosts achievement. Curiosity can expand our empathy, when we are curious about others and talk to people. Interesting, isn't it?

Favourite Food Thought 'C':
- *Celery juice!*

Celery juice has been widely hailed as a miraculous superfood, with an incredible ability to create sweeping improvements for all kinds of health issues. I have seen first-hand the power of celery to cure many skin ailments and liver issues, and to detoxify the system. It's also very low-calorie and has a particular taste that makes it versatile in many recipes. I drink carrot, apple and celery juice myself to self-cure and as a health tonic. And did you know that if you cut the end off a bunch of celery and place it in water, the celery will grow and you can snip it and have it as a microgreen on your meals?

You might also like to check out this website (belonging to Anthony William, a chronic illness expert and the originator of the global celery juice movement – he's also the host of the 'Medical Medium' podcast and the author of several bestselling books) to explore how celery juice could be good for you:
https://www.medicalmedium.com/medical-medium-celery-juice-movement

D.   'D' IS FOR 'DO YOUR BEST'

A job well done can lead to great satisfaction.

Do your best, for that is all you can do. Doing your best can bring you great success and add to your happiness.

Three important things to remember:
- Make sure that whatever you do, you really apply yourself and give it your best.
- You can actually do whatever you want or like, providing it causes no harm anywhere.
- The old adage is true:-
    Good, better, best;
    Never let it rest,
    Until your good is better,
    And your better is the best!

Garden Tip 'D':
- *Dung!*

Yes, dung! It was one of Dad's favourite things! Now I say that tongue-in-cheek, but manure is actually the secret to wonderful plant growth, for we all need nourishment and fertilising, don't we? Dad used to keep chickens and he would scoop their pen floors and make a liquid fertiliser. He would also go hunting for dry cowpats out in the paddocks – these were put in a hessian bag and crunched up and sprinkled by hand onto the garden dry (using gardening gloves, of course!), and then hosed in with water.

Natural Therapy Thought 'D':
- *Dandruff remedy.*

To combat that annoying itching and the unsightly shoulder snow, both topical and internal remedies can be used. Topically, use a hot olive oil pack, or vitamin E, or rosemary oil, or a nettle tea rinse. Internally, take essential fatty acids and rosemary oil. I find these are magic!

Favourite Food Thought 'D':
- *Dandelion tea.*

I have always been a big fan of dandelion tea. The over-the-counter tea from Bonvit is a great coffee substitute, and the Symingtons dandelion beverage is also amazing, but making it yourself is a lot of fun too. You can buy organic dandelion root, or the dehydrated dandelion leaf. Or you can even forage it yourself.

I have loved the book **Eat Weeds** by Diego Bonetto from the moment I opened it, as it 'opened my plant eyes' further! I suggest you purchase a copy if you are keen on foraging – it will guide you in how to forage, identify and harvest your target plants. To find and use the dandelion, you have to be able to recognise the dandelion!

To use dandelion root, dig it up, break off the aerial leaves, wash it well, slice it up, and leave it to dry on an oven tray. Turn the oven on and let it heat up empty. Turn the oven off, add the tray of sliced root, close the door and leave overnight. The next morning the product is dehydrated and ready to use how you choose. For dandelion root tea, place a spoonful of dried dandelion root in a small teapot and add boiling water and let it steep for ten minutes. Dandelion leaves can also be dehydrated like this and used in a similar way to make a variation on the tea.

You're welcome!

E.   'E' IS FOR 'EAT GOOD FOOD'

Eat good food, and eat less food.

Many of us overeat and even children today can struggle with obesity. Make sure you eat only as much as your body needs. Cut down on portion sizes, and make sure that whatever you eat is healthy, wholesome, fresh food. If the food you eat isn't supporting your health, don't eat it.

Three important things to remember:
- Choose healthy styles of cooking and use mostly fresh and wholesome food.
- Try using smaller plates with smaller serves, and eat slowly.
- Keep special treats for special occasions.

Garden Tip 'E':
- *Edible.*

Grow as many edible things as you can.

I have many fond childhood memories of identifying and harvesting fruit, vegetables and herbs for the table. Likewise my own daughter, and similarly my grandchildren, too. So much knowledge also to impart and share about just the joy of nature, sunshine, and water – simple joys in simple things that now I feel in modern-day society may have largely gone out the window.

There aren't really many excuses for not being able to grow something – you can grow things in patio pots and even on the windowsill if needed. I'll share with you my tips for growing herbs in patio pots. Choose a large-enough pot and a good growing soil. Choose a sunny location, and water well and regularly. Don't over-fertilise. Do harvest often!

If you really can't grow it yourself, you can always support local 'grandpa and grandma' growers, local farmers (farmers' markets are treasure-troves), and roadside stalls – fresh is best.

Natural Therapy Thought 'E':
- *Earache remedy.*

You can use eardrops of mullein oil, OR myrrh oil, OR fresh parsley juice (perhaps from parsley you have grown yourself?). Internally, supplements that may help include vitamin A, vitamin C, zinc, magnesium, and garlic.

Favourite Food Thought 'E':
- *Eggs.*

I think that the best protein is the egg!

Some of my favourite foods that use eggs are: English quiche, frittata, Spanish eggs, soy sauce pickled eggs, souffle, angel food cake, velveting chicken, royal icing, lemon curd, devilled eggs with caviar, and hard-boiled eggs as a salad topping.

How hungry are you getting right now?

Besides the edible recipes, you can also use eggshells (all crunched up) in the garden, and eggshells smashed into grit to feed the chickens. And a lovely non-food one is to use a mixture of egg and oatmeal and honey as a facial mask.

I have so many fond memories of making ALL of the abovementioned over the past 80 years of my life, notably the fun nourishing masks with my daughter, and gifting the lemon curd to many people. I've been told that my lemon curd is everyone's favourite gift to receive from me, other than my hugs!

I'm sure Google will help you out with recipes for any of the above, but if you specifically want any of my family recipes, please reach out (see page 89 of this book) – I'm happy to share.

F. 'F' IS FOR 'FUN IS YOUR FRIEND'

Fun in life is most important – make sure you find it!

Develop a positive attitude and seek out things that you enjoy doing. Join like-minded friends in hobbies, outings and enjoyable activities.

Three important things to remember:
- Make sure you find your fun – we all need it.
- Fun 'joins in' when you do the things you like.
- Invest in entertainment such as clubs, hobbies, sports, or other fun pastimes – it's all there for you to enjoy.

Garden Tip 'F':
- *Fences.*

Just because there is a fence on your property, don't let that hinder your growing prowess. Use the FENCE space. Over the years I have used fences for things such as passionfruit and trailing beans. I even wound the jasmine around my fence and made a jasmine wall, to the envy of most neighbours. "Why didn't we think of that?" they chorused.

Natural Therapy Thought 'F':
- *Flower essence therapy.*

This is a type of therapy that uses liquid essences of flowers to promote emotional, spiritual and physical wellbeing. Flowers are soaked in water that is then heated and filtered (some alcohol may be added at the end as a preservative), retaining only the natural liquid energy and essence of the flowers. Flower essences can be ingested or applied topically (those who are pregnant or breastfeeding should choose essences without alcohol), and have been reported to improve mood and relieve pain. You may even already know of Bach's Rescue Remedy (see also the 'T' section of this chapter), which is a popular flower essence combination that many people have been happily using since it was developed over 80 years ago. I certainly love it, but my favourites would have to be the Australian Bush Flower Essences, which I like to use to help dispel any mind-body aggravations that might try to hamper my happiness.

Favourite Recipe 'F':
- *French!*

French foods and the French language rate very high on my happiness dial. I have travelled extensively most of my adult life. I learned French as a second language and have participated in many conversations over the years. As far as French food goes, I am not a fan of garlic, any fatty or jellied meats, pork, shellfish or liver. However, I do love duck, all things soups, and all things vegetables (especially artichokes). I also love eggs many ways, particularly omelettes. And of course, I absolutely love crêpes Suzette – those delicately thin pancakes with a delicious buttery liqueur sauce.

Happiness is crêpes Suzette!

INGREDIENTS, CRÊPES

- Eggs, 2 large
- All-purpose flour, *3/4* cup
- Whole milk, *1/2* cup
- Sugar, *1/2* teaspoon
- Cold water, *1/3* cup
- Oil, 1 tablespoon
- Unsalted butter, 1 tablespoon

INGREDIENTS, SAUCE

- Unsalted butter, *1/2* cup
- Granulated sugar, *1/3* cup
- Fine orange zest, *1/2* teaspoon
- Flavoured liqueur of choice (see METHOD, SAUCE), 3 tablespoons
- Cognac, 1 tablespoon
- Extra sugar to sprinkle

METHOD, CRÊPES

- Whisk eggs, flour, and whole milk in a bowl until smooth.
- Whisk into the same bowl the sugar, cold water, oil, and the (melted and cooled) unsalted butter.
- Heat a 10-inch crêpe pan over medium heat. Pour the batter into the pan to make a thin covering. Wait until the shine on the crêpe's surface has gone and the crêpe curls a little, and then flip and cook the other side briefly. Stack the cooked crêpes on a warm plate as you repeat the cooking process for the whole batter amount.

METHOD, SAUCE

- Carefully and slowly heat in a flat pan until bubbling (stirring occasionally) a mixture of the unsalted butter, granulated sugar, orange zest, and two tablespoons of your chosen liqueur (Grand Marnier or Cointreau orange liqueur, or Tia Maria if you prefer coffee over orange flavour).

- When the sauce is ready, take each warm crêpe, fold it into a triangle shape, dip it in the sauce to cover, and then arrange it in the pan. Continue until all crêpes are contained in the pan of sauce.

- Sprinkle a little extra sugar over the surface of the crêpes arrangement, then pour over a mixture of one tablespoon of your chosen liqueur plus one tablespoon of cognac. Ignite the alcohol, wait for the flame to die down, then serve the crêpes immediately.

G.   'G' IS FOR 'GIVE, AND GIVE WILLINGLY'

Giving adds to the happiness of both the giver and the receiver.

Giving is an important part of life. It is so very rewarding that by giving, the happiness of both the giver and receiver is increased. Make sure that you give willingly, and without the expectation of receiving anything in return. Nevertheless, you will find that the more you give out, the more you will get back.

Three important things to remember:
- Be a generous giver – the more giving, the more receiving.
- Be positive about giving.
- Beware of what you give, because if you give out negativity, you will receive negativity in return.

Garden Tip 'G':
- *Gardening itself!*

I couldn't live without a garden; it's simply LIFE to me.

The best gardening tip I have is to grow something you LOVE, because then you will be passionate about it, nurture it and enjoy the rewards. It's like children with seeds. It doesn't matter what plant it is; they enjoy planting the seeds, watering them, watching the tiny green shoots emerge from the soil and watching each leaf sprout – that's it.

My daughter loved to grow edible seeds. I'd get alfalfa, mung, wheat and barley and place them in a jar together. For about one-eighth of a jar of seeds, place a nylon stocking over one end and put in water. Rinse the seeds daily and place the jar in a dark cupboard, and repeat. In a few days the seeds would sprout and in another couple of days we had edible sprouts and seeds for our salads. So much fun!

Natural Therapy Thought 'G':
- *For care of your gums.*

I have lots of experience in this area!

For relief of sore gums I can use any of the following: sage tea, rosehip tea, tea tree oil, vitamin B complex, vitamin C, gelsemium, yarrow, arnica, or ferrum phos homeopathics.

A twice-daily treatment using turmeric powder and salt water also promotes fast healing in the case of gingivitis, helping to reduce swelling and inflammation and assist repair of your gums. Take a quarter teaspoon of turmeric powder and mix with water until you make a paste. Apply to the affected gums for five minutes and rub with gentle massaging motions. Rinse off with salt water.

Favourite Food Thought 'G':
- *Grapefruit.*

I was introduced to this delightful fruit many years ago. Two of my uncles grew the most juicy grapefruit – both the pink and yellow kinds – and it became something of a family tradition to share and eat them. These days I can no longer eat them, due to being on blood pressure medication, but my memories of them are divine and to be celebrated.

On a family Fiji visit, my husband and daughter and I had the best HUGE – as large as dinner plates! – pink grapefruits we had ever eaten. We each enjoyed half a grapefruit, prepared for us in segments, with no need for any sprinkled sugar on top. Upon our return to Melbourne, I asked our daughter what she would like for breakfast. "GRAPEFRUIT, of course!" she responded, and that's how our obsession started.

And each Christmas, we would have so much fun! My husband and I would pack one of my nylon stockings full of goodies for our daughter to wake up to on Christmas morning. I could stretch that nylon from under the Christmas tree, along the hallway, through the kitchen and back again – imagine how many things I was able to fit in it! A can of baked beans, a book, apples, so many little Christmas gifts, bags of nuts to crack, and...PINK GRAPEFRUITS! So many fond and citrusy memories.

H.   'H' IS FOR 'HAVE A GOAL'

Work enthusiastically on your goals and you will succeed with joy.

Having a goal can boost your happiness by encouraging you to focus on what you enjoy, and enable you to derive joy from your success. Joy adds to happiness!

Three important things to remember:
- Having a goal sets you on a path.
- Decide what you want and how to get it, then aim for it with passion and clarity!
- Thoroughly enjoy the trip of working towards your goal.

Garden Tip 'H':
- *Herbs!*

PLANT THEM!
USE THEM!
ENJOY THEM!
That is all I can really say here, without needing a whole extra book to extol all the virtues of herbs – as food, as food enhancement, as medicine, as insect repellent, as therapy, as mood boosters, as objects of beauty in their own right...the list goes on and on...
If you invest in a herb garden in some form, even if it is just a handful of

pots on your kitchen windowsill, you will be so very glad!

Natural Therapy Thought 'H':
- *Handmade cards.*

My love for handmade things extended into card-making, and pressing the flowers I grew in my garden in a flower press and creating wonderful gifts for people. I have been blessed with the artistic flair, and to be honest, I just love creating! I think it's a wonderful thing, to invent mini pieces of art, to spread joy and allow others to experience joy too. It's warming to me to see the glint of happiness in someone's eyes when you give them a gift. I love lifting my mood and relieving stress, and spreading the sense of joy to those who receive my cards. The extra personal touch that comes from something handmade enriches me as much as it enriches the recipient of my creativity and love. I think I have to go and make some cards now! It's an age-old craft, expressed from when we were young children. I'm sure you have all received a handmade item from a child, and relished the moment? And of course I love getting cards too, that others have taken the time to handmake for me. It can make my day, or even my week, to receive a card from a loved one in the post.

Favourite Recipe 'H':
- *Haricot bean hummus.*

My father, I'm sure, wouldn't have had it any other way than for me to mention Scotland's signature dish, HAGGIS. However, I'm not going to go into any detail as I've never approved of this Scottish table food icon. Sorry, Dad!

I might have focussed on HONEY instead – also nature's antibiotic and skin replenisher – except that sadly I can't eat it as I have been allergic to it all my life.

But third time lucky, because HARICOT BEANS will get some love here. These small whitish-coloured beans are also called navy beans, Boston beans, or white peas. They have a buttery texture and are a great source of protein (similar to cannellini beans), making them perfect for casseroles, soups, and salads. YUM!

Try my easy haricot bean hummus (without garlic, as I'm allergic to that too!).

INGREDIENTS AND METHOD

- Rinse and drain a 400 g can of haricot beans (if you want to use dried beans instead, boil water and soak them overnight, rinsing them once).
- In a blender, add the beans and dribble in a good quality oil, about two tablespoons per can or dried/soaked equivalent of beans.
- Run the blender for three minutes or until the mixture is smooth.
- Add the juice of one lemon, two tablespoons of tahini, and a pinch each of salt and pepper. Add a pinch of paprika if so desired.
- Scoop your hummus out of the blender and serve.

I. 'I' IS FOR 'INVEST IN A SMILE'

Smiles are contagious.

Investing in a smile is most advantageous and can add to the happiness of all present. When you smile, others often follow suit, and this can change the whole atmosphere!

Three important things to remember:
- When you smile you feel good, and when another person smiles at you, you both feel good!
- If you see someone without a smile, give them one of yours.
- A room full of smiling faces is a very happy place.

Garden Tip 'I':
- *Igloo!*

I mean a garden igloo, or bubble-house, or hothouse! I did housesitting for many years, and so many of the homes had sunrooms – essentially hothouses for the owners' vegetables and orchids and other flowers; being in them was just bliss. Not only was each place a waterproof balcony or porch, but it was a true delight to see the flowers and vegetables all sharing the same space. The gatherer in me enjoyed the harvesting all year round, too! I have been told it's now a 'glamping experience' to camp out in a sunhouse, or 'sun igloo' – how fun and joyous!

Natural Therapy Thought 'I':
- *Combatting indigestion.*

Indigestion has plagued every single member of our family for as long as I can recall. Chewing on dried grapefruit peel helps. Also try a linseed oil and meadowsweet poultice. Eating aniseed and fennel may help; also Irish moss. You can also take digestive enzymes, lactobacillus, or white chestnut. The homeopathic supplements sodium phosphate (Nat Phos) and magnesium phosphate (Mag Phos) may also help.

Favourite Recipe 'I':
- *Italian seasoning.*

Specifically, my homemade Italian seasoning. I use it for flavouring chicken, soups, pizzas, and a variety of other savoury dishes. I also keep some in a salt shaker for table use, too.

INGREDIENTS AND METHOD
- Basil, basil, basil! Yes, I love basil!
- Parsley, parsley, parsley! Yes, I love parsley even more!
- Oregano.
- Rosemary.
- A touch of thyme, when I feel like it. All of these are out of my garden, of course (see also section 'H' in this chapter!).
- Harvest all of the chosen herbs, wash and dry them, and lay them on oven trays.
- Preheat the oven, then turn it off. Insert the herb trays quickly, close the oven door, and leave things overnight.
- In the morning, remove the trays from the oven.
- As applicable, destalk the leaves from any too-large stalks. Use a mortar

and pestle to grind the retained leaves and small stalks to a fine powder. VOILÀ!

J. 'J' IS FOR 'JOIN A GROUP'

Happiness thrives on joint adventures.

Joining a group is a great way to expand your happiness. Happiness grows with new friends, new interests, and new places. You can choose what you want to do and share it with others who enjoy it too.

Three important things to remember:
- Link up with like-minded people.
- Group support encourages 'getting out and about' to do what you enjoy.
- Happiness increases when you share activities and adventures with friends.

Garden Tip 'J':
- *Jacaranda.*

The jacaranda has always been a favourite of mine. We lived for several years in a beautiful home in Ringwood, Victoria, and our jacaranda tree was lush with its magnificent purple pyramidal blooms each spring. It kept its foliage all year round and we would have little picnics under it. Its elegance was delightful. If you have some space and a bright sunny location with sun all day, it's a great low-maintenance tree to have, and it attracts many birds, too. I fondly remember the blue wrens and willie wagtails who would come and sit at our picnics!

Natural Therapy Thought 'J':
- *Relief of joint pain.*

Skin-brushing and using a loofah in hot water, and applying heat packs, have all helped me over the advancing years. Willow tea is also wonderful as both a tonic and refreshing drink.

Favourite Food Thought 'J':
- *Jam.*

I come from a long line of gardeners, harvesters, cooks, and preservers. I am renowned in my circle of family and friends for the preserves I make, and chief among them is jam. The satisfaction of making, and gifting, and eating the jam I make, and seeing others loving to eat the jam I make especially for them (some people like conserves, some prefer jellies, and all in between), certainly makes me happy!
And how WONDERFUL my kitchen smells on my jam-making days!

K.   'K' IS FOR 'KEEP PERSEVERING'

If you wish to succeed, you need to persevere.

You know that Rome wasn't built in a day. It takes time and patience to achieve worthwhile things, especially if you are pursuing a goal after you have found a new focus or changed your attitude. Make sure that you encourage yourself to persevere with the 'new you' so you can achieve your happiness.

Three important things to remember:
- Lazy effort often leads to failure, so make sure that you really apply yourself and persist.
- Keep persevering with your changed attitude to bring about a change to your happiness.
- Keep telling yourself: "It's something I need to BE and it's something I need to FEEL."

Garden Tip 'K':
- *Keep on keeping the pests at bay!*

Every gardener is plagued by garden pests – aphids on roses, fruit tree scale insects, earwigs, thrips, caterpillars (Mother waged constant war against cabbage white butterfly caterpillars in particular), harlequin bugs, slugs, snails (or 'shellbacks' as Mother used to call them!)… They all want a piece of the garden that is being carefully cultivated by and for the humans. What can we do about them?

When I was a child, the family would go out at night with lights and buckets to pluck the little creatures off the plants; we also used tissues to squash what was squashable! I continued to do this a lot over the years, including in the gardens I had as an adult, especially as I don't like to use the commercial chemical insect repellents and killers.

Dad did have another way to deal with the pests naturally, though – he swore by a concoction of garlic, chillies, and dish detergent, which he dispensed onto the plants with a spray bottle. It was an across-the-board pest-killer that didn't harm the plants or the humans, with the wonderful bonus that Mother and I got to escape the bucket-filler and tissue-squisher duties!

Natural Therapy Thought 'K':
- *K is for potassium.*

Yes, really! 'K' is the chemical symbol for potassium (from its Latin name, *kalium*). Most people know that potassium is necessary for regulating blood pressure, but it has so many other biological functions that are crucial for our health. Fortunately for us, our potassium requirements can be met through a diet of natural food, as potassium is found in so many vegetables and fruits. It's very much a situation of 'a banana a day keeps the doctor away' – except that it would be more like 11 bananas!

> **WARNING: FOR PEOPLE WITH KIDNEY DISEASE.**
> People with kidney disease should not consume potassium-rich foods or potassium supplements – please check with your doctor

if this is or could be you.

Favourite Food Thought 'K':
- *Kale.*

This is a 'superfood' that I have loved since I was a child, long before it was fashionable. Of course Dad grew kale – curly kale, Chinese kale, black kale – in his incredible vegetable garden, and it was my favourite of all the green vegetables. I remember when we had to soak and soak the harvested curly kale in salt water in the laundry tub, to dislodge the earwigs that loved to hide in the leaves! But then the leaves were all ours, and how versatile they were, too. I loved kale by itself, or in salads and soups – you can use it everywhere you'd use spinach. Whenever I eat it now I feel like it's giving me a warm hug, and I'm thrilled about its new popularity of today.

L.   'L' IS FOR 'LEARN TO LOVE TO BE HAPPY'

Love your own happiness.

Love and enjoy your own happiness, rather than envying others. Don't allow circumstances and daily happenings to bring you down. You can rise above them all and succeed, when you love being happy!

Three important things to remember:
- Don't get bogged down wallowing in misery, but instead make sure that you want HAPPINESS.
- Knowing that you can be happy lets you enjoy being happy.
- When you love being happy, others will also love you for it.

Garden Tip 'L':
- *Lemon aid.*

Lemons! They are just so useful – as food, as medicine, as a natural cleaner, as a pest repellent, and more…they can even be used in soap-making. To me, a garden without a lemon tree feels incomplete. Even if you don't have space for a mini-orchard, it's possible to grow a little lemon tree in a patio pot. Place in a sunny spot and ensure good drainage, do just a little pruning to keep the height down, and do some 'decongesting' to encourage bushiness. Combat pests with designs on your lemons by using Dad's natural garlic/chillies/detergent concoction (see section 'K' in this chapter).

Natural Therapy Thought 'L':
- *Lemons against liver spots.*

Surprise! Now we can use some (maybe home-grown) lemons to combat liver spots on the skin. Simply apply lemon juice directly to the liver spots, then go enjoy some time in the sunshine.

Favourite Recipe 'L':
- *Lemon butter syrup cake.*

After your success in growing your own lemons (and perhaps after having treated your liver spots!), there's nothing that says celebration quite like a cake. This cake is an easy one that my daughter makes for any occasion. You'll need some pre-made lemon curd (either homemade or store-bought) and an appetite for sour sweetness!

INGREDIENTS
- Lemons, 2
- Lemon curd, 3 tablespoons
- Fine sugar, 1 cup for the cake plus 3 tablespoons for the syrup
- Eggs, 3
- Butter, 4 large knobs (melted and cooled)
- Self-raising flour, 3 cups

METHOD
- Zest and juice one lemon and place the zest and juice in a bowl.
- Add the cup of sugar, the eggs, the lemon curd and the butter, and mix well with a spoon.

- Add the flour and mix well with a spoon.
- Bake the mixture in a lined tin at 180 degrees Celsius for 30 minutes or until a skewer comes out clean.
- In a cup, place the juice and half the zest of the second lemon, add the three tablespoons of sugar, and mix well to make a syrup.
- Spoon the syrup over the hot cake, and serve immediately – yum yum!

M.   'M' IS FOR 'MOVE OFTEN AND KEEP MOVING'

Move, and move it, and do it now!

Too many people wait around for happiness to come to them. They may have a very long wait! So rather than waiting, get moving. Actively generate your own happiness by moving your mind and body to create what you enjoy. Again, don't wait – do it now!

Three important things to remember:
- Don't sit around and wait for happiness to join you.
- Move yourself and work on it, because only you can make you happy.
- There is no room for laziness – do it now!

Garden Tip 'M':
- *Mother's love of dahlias.*

Mother had a great love for gardening, and for dahlias in particular, so this section is about them, and dedicated to her.

The bushy, tuberous perennials of many and varied kinds of dahlias adorned the front garden of Mother's home. They were real showstoppers and were entered in many competitions in the local community. The flowers would be picked and taken to the church and the local hall, featuring as the centrepiece at many community functions. I have memories of earwigs nestling in the petals and scaring the people who found them!

Mother was born in September 1914 at Clonbinane in country Victoria, and attended school at Sunday Creek. She was the embodiment of MOVING. She told us stories of walking herself and all of her many younger siblings to school and home again; that would take hours. There were also hours of assisting her own mother with the housework, cooking and child-rearing. She was the embodiment of DOING IT ALL (must be generational!). Later she lived in Nyora where she spent her early adult years working at boarding houses and hotels. She then met and married Dad, who at the time was a fettler (conducting repairs on the country railways) and a woodcutter. My parents eventually retired to Broadford, where their magnificent gardens continued to be nurtured. Dad died in 1988, and Mother passed away when she was 83.

For maximised dahlia flower production in the summer, propagate and pinch the dahlia plants. Early in the season, do high-nitrogen fertilising and composting, and stake the dahlias at this time immediately after planting. Continue to tie them up during their growth cycle. A regular watering schedule is vital also – do deep watering three times a week as opposed to a quick water daily. Pinch at the top of the plants to take off the uppermost leaves. The plants will fill out and give you more flowers for the full season. Pinch off the spent/dead blooms at the stem.

Natural Therapy Thought 'M':
- *Massage.*

I am a great fan of bodywork, and have been for most of my life. It has saved me from pain and injury, and aided my recovery from injury, disease, and stress. It has inspired me to study it myself as I did for many years, and became a large part of my working career too. I have many many massage books from the 1960s, '70s, and '80s – to me they are of medicinal value and in my opinion should be studied like medicine. I'm very glad my daughter also thought this – she has been a medical massage and injury management specialist for many years now, as well as a homeopathic physician. So all of this information is backed by science, by me and my 60 years of experience and expertise, and by my daughter too, Dr. Dee.

Favourite Food Thought 'M':
- *Minestrone.*

Minestrone is one of my favourite soups to make, to eat and to serve to others too. It's the best chunky soup in the world! And the beauty of it is you can customise it to exactly your own taste, allergies and nutrition preferences by mixing up the types and combinations of meat, beans, chunky vegetables and pasta. You can find any number of recipes online to suit exactly what you'd like – just remember that there will be a lot of chopping involved, and it has to be CHUNKY! I like it with freshly grated parmesan cheese and some of my own homemade sourdough bread.

N.   'N' IS FOR 'NEEDS'

Be aware of your needs for happiness.

If you are unhappy, you need to work on yourself to identify and change the things that need changing for you to achieve being happy. Surround yourself with support while you change, including by interacting and doing things with others who are happy.

Three important things to remember:
- Be aware of your need to act.
- You need to seek out activities that make you happy.
- Interact with other happy people.

Garden Tip 'N':
- *Nettles in the garden.*

Dad used to go and pull all the stinging nettles out of the garden. One day I went and helped him, because they were growing like weeds. Dad pulled so many nettles that the pile (which we later burned) was a couple of feet off the ground, but he never complained. Well, I pulled one nettle, and I screamed! They are called 'stinging nettles' for a reason! Dad then showed me the secret of how to 'deal with the stingers'. The stingers were on top of the bush to ward off things that would eat the plants, so by grabbing the bush from underneath, you simply didn't get stung.

When nettles were becoming popular in the 1970s and '80s for their food and medicinal uses, we stopped weeding nettles and started harvesting them instead. My daughter would join in the harvesting then too, helping Grandad, who by then was providing nettles (and a vast array of other vegetables) to the local grocer shops of Broadford. The store owners and customers would ask how we picked the nettles, and would say that we were very brave. We never had nettle rashes and everyone thought we must have worn some VERY sturdy gardening gloves!

Natural Therapy Thought 'N':
- *Nettles as medicine.*

Nettles can assist in the treatment of hypertension, diabetes and allergies. They make a good blood thinner and diuretic, and are a good source of lithium to help you sleep. They can be taken as supplements, eaten as a vegetable, or steeped to make a tea.

Favourite Food Thought 'N':
- *Nettles as food.*

Once you remove the sting (by pouring hot water over the nettles, or by cooking, crushing or drying them), you can use nettles in a variety of foods. I like them in stews, smoothies, stir-fries and salads, but my favourite use for them is in soup.

You can sauté nettles in butter as for any leafy vegetable, and then add them as a component vegetable to any soup you like. Or you can make nettles the hero of your soup. Classic nettle soup involves taking a few chopped potatoes, a couple of chopped celery stalks, your chosen liquid stock, chopped onion/leek, some prepared nettles, and your favourite herbs and seasonings. Simply cook until the vegetables are tender, and then blend until smooth. Delicious!

O.   'O' IS FOR 'OPEN UP'

You need to openly admit you are unhappy before you can change.

Once you have opened up and acknowledged that you are unhappy and recognised that you want to change, you are ready to make a start to work on yourself and your goal of achieving happiness. Then don't hesitate – do it now! Change your negative thinking, be optimistic, and believe and KNOW you can be happy.

Three important things to remember:
- Don't be afraid to open up and admit you are not happy.
- Change your attitude and work on happiness.
- Be optimistic and enthusiastic about creating your change.

Garden Tip 'O':
- *Please your 'oeil'.*

Trompe-l'oeil (pronounced 'trom-ploy'), French for 'deceive the eye', is a term describing flat art or fixtures that give the sense of an optical illusion of depth. One of the most beautiful home gardens I ever saw belonged to a retired army officer and his wife for whom I would sometimes housesit. Their garden was small but it was magnificent, and it included a *trompe-l'oeil* feature with a mirror beyond it that created an extra 'dimension' to their garden. Here I would sit in the sun, drinking my tea, and quietly enjoying life.

My point is that while the main heart and soul of a garden will always be its plants, there may also be a place for non-biological contents that can really elevate, personalise and beautify your garden space.

Open your mind to looking at possibilities with a new set of eyes, for pleasing your eye.

Natural Therapy Thought 'O':
- *The oldest therapy.*

I'm talking about ayurveda, an ancient philosophy of medicine and therapy from India. I have applied ayurvedic knowledge and practices throughout my life, including physical therapies, rituals, herbs, tinctures and massage. A very dear friend of mine (whom I speak of in more detail in section '9' in the next chapter) used to take annual trips to India, and each time she would bring back many treasures of ayurvedic information and items, that to this day continue to help and inspire me in my life.

Favourite Recipe 'O':
- *Out-of-this-world hummingbird cake.*

This is my daughter's hummingbird cake recipe, and I think it's the best I've ever had, so kudos to her! From the batter mixture she makes three small cakes, then sandwiches them together with the pineapple cream cheese frosting to result in a single stacked cake.

Beware – the finished cake will not last long, because hungry mouths will gobble it up!

INGREDIENTS
- VERY ripe bananas, 3
- Can of crushed pineapple (440 g) or half a fresh pineapple, puréed (fresh is best if you can get it), plus one extra cup of canned or fresh pineapple pieces
- Eggs, 4
- Oil, 2 tablespoons
- Chopped mixed nuts (your choice of pecans, hazelnuts, walnuts), 1 cup (optional), plus extra for decoration (optional)
- Sugar, 1 cup
- Lemon, 1
- Maple syrup or honey, *1/4* cup
- Self-raising flour, 2&*1/2* cups

- Cinnamon (optional)
- Cream cheese, 250 g block
- Icing sugar (AKA powdered sugar; amount as needed)

METHOD
- Mash the bananas well, beat the eggs, and juice the lemon. Set a dash of the lemon juice aside for later use.
- In a large bowl, place all of the mashed bananas, the crushed/puréed pineapple, the beaten eggs, the oil, the cup of chopped nuts (if using), the sugar, the majority of the lemon juice, and the maple syrup (or honey). Mix well.
- Add the flour, and cinnamon to taste (if using). Mix well.
- Divide the batter between three small lined cake tins. Bake 20 minutes at 180 degrees Celsius, or until skewers come out clean.
- Turn the cakes out onto a rack and allow them to cool while you make the pineapple cream cheese frosting.
- In a new bowl, warm and soften the cream cheese. Add the cup of pineapple pieces (retain some pieces for final decoration, if desired) and the dash of lemon juice, and mix.
- Add whatever quantity of icing/powdered sugar is required to get the desired frosting taste and consistency. The frosting needs to be thick enough to support the sandwiching of the three cakes without the layers sliding apart.
- Use most of the frosting between the layers to build the stacked cake. Reserve some of the frosting for the top of the cake. Decorate the top of the cake with additional mixed nuts, pineapple pieces, and/or cinnamon, if desired. Enjoy!

P.   'P' IS FOR 'PLEASE BE POLITE'

Being polite will create allies of those around you.

It is important to get people 'on your side', to find the smoothest way through life and to promote happiness in yourself and others. But getting people on-side does not mean being pushy or bullying! When you are polite, gentle, persuasive and agreeable, you will attract similar attributes in others. Similar-minded people can then all work together on happiness for all – everyone will benefit and there will be happy times for all.

Three important things to remember:
- It is to your advantage to develop a polite frame of mind.
- Approach happiness with gentle persuasion.
- Similar-minded people attracted to one another will help one another.

Garden Tip 'P':
- *Patience!*

I have always had a lot of patience, which is a great asset when tending a garden. Patience to wait for the plants to grow, to wait for the sun to shine again, to wait for the rain to fall, to wait for the fruit and vegetables to ripen or be harvest-ready. All of it. Plant it and it will grow, nurture it and it will produce, wait and the fruits will ripen. Remember to enjoy the entire PROCESS, not just the end results.

Natural Therapy Thought 'P':
- *Pets.*

I am sure this will be news to no one who shares their home with a companion animal, but pets are so good for us! Pets benefit both our physical and mental health. It may be that a cat's purr vibrates at the right frequency to help heal our injuries and ailments, or simply that the act of caring for and about a dog or rabbit or goldfish decreases stress and promotes heart health. We had a beautiful little black poodle, Princess Pompy, as our family dog for many years. And when I was housesitting for many more years after that, there were so many little 'loaner' pet friends to love.

Pets are happiness-givers and happiness-receivers, and I feel blessed for the memories of every darling animal I have known in my life.

Favourite Food Thought 'P':
- *Peaches.*

I have many fond memories of visiting local stone fruit orchards and buying cases of apricots, nectarines and peaches. The fruit that actually made it home then went into all manner of delicious desserts. This recipe at Well Plated online will really give you a taste of one of our absolute family favourites, baked peaches:
https://www.wellplated.com/baked-peaches/

Q.   'Q' IS FOR 'QUEUE UP FOR HUGS'

Hugs are the simplest pieces of happiness to give and receive.

The feeling you get from giving or receiving a hug says 'happiness', so they are very important. Hugs are food for the soul! An ancient guru once said, "Eight hugs a day should be the minimum." They do really work to promote happiness and wellbeing. And do you want to know something wonderful? Everybody hugs in the same language!

Three important things to remember:
- Hugs feed the soul – join the 'Q'!
- The feeling you get from a hug says: "Happiness is here."
- Hugs really work for happiness, so hug often!

Garden Tip 'Q':
- *Queuing for information.*

Dad seemed to know a lot about gardening almost simply by instinct, but he was always keen to pick up new information where he could. He thought very highly of the Old Farmer's Almanac, and each new edition we managed to acquire would quickly be read cover-to-cover. These days

it's very easy to access the Old Farmer's Almanac online, and I can't recommend it highly enough for anyone with an interest in gardening, from beginners to experts:
https://www.almanac.com/

Natural Therapy Thought 'Q':
- *Quinine.*

I think that quinine is a little miracle, especially in the treatment of malaria, to help curb the cyclic nature of occurrence of malarial fever and chills. In tropical North Queensland, my daughter also uses it in the treatment of Ross River fever and Barmah Forest virus infection, along with its homeopathic use in the treatment of gout and rheumatism.

Favourite Food Thought 'Q':
- *Quince jelly.*

I love quinces, and I am renowned for my quince jelly. But rather than write out my own recipe here, I'm going to refer you to a cooking blog website called Fuss Free Flavours, where there is a quince jelly recipe so similar to mine that I couldn't help but wonder if its creator and I were psychically connected…at least where quinces were concerned!

So please enjoy this delicious recipe, which is accompanied by extra titbits of information and beautiful progress photos to illustrate the process:
https://fussfreeflavours.com/how-to-make-quince-jelly/

R. 'R' IS FOR 'REASON TO LIVE'

Your reason for living should also be your reason to be happy.

If you are unhappy in your life, change your reasoning and work on achieving your happiness. To live happily is your goal! Work on it with all you have, and make it happen. Your reason for living and your reason to be happy go together when you decide to make it so.

Three important things to remember:
- When you have a reason to live you have a reason to be happy.
- Make your reason for living work for you to achieve and increase your happiness.
- Decide to be happy – it is up to you.

Garden Tip 'R':
- *Reduce your stress.*

Quite simply, gardening can make you feel more peaceful and content. Focussing your attention on the immediate tasks and details of gardening can reduce negative thoughts and feelings and make you feel amazing in the exact moment. Just spending time around plants, out in nature, in the sunshine and breeze, simply outdoors, eases stress for many.

Natural Therapy Thought 'R':
- *Rash treatment.*

There are many things that can be used to help soothe a rash. Check online or with your natural medicine practitioner about whether the following may be useful for you.

Chickweed ointment can be used topically, as can soda water. Irish moss, cold/heat application, aloe vera juice, red clover tea, diluted apple cider vinegar, rose oil, celery juice, and cucumber juice (both for drinking and for topical application) have all been reported to have helped.

On a different rash note, and thinking of apple cider vinegar, I do have a funny story to tell! My father loved vinegar, and he brewed his own apple cider vinegar from the little snow apples that he and Mother grew. He would often open the tap of the brewing barrel and take a long drink from it direct. "Mmm, lassie, delicious!" he said to me once, in his thick Scottish accent. Encouraged by this endorsement and being a trusting small child at the time, I followed his example and took a sip of the vinegar myself. I spluttered it everywhere! I couldn't believe how awful it was, and I was shocked that Dad just drank it like it was sweet apple juice!

Favourite Recipe 'R':
- *Relish the relish!*

My 'famous' New Zealand sweet tomato relish is what I consider my best recipe. It has been consumed by our family for over 50 years, and has also delighted our many friends and acquaintances who have received it as gifts.

INGREDIENTS
- Very ripe tomatoes, 750 g
- Onions, 600 g
- Apples, 2
- Vinegar (white or brown), 300 ml
- Raw sugar, 300 g
- Cornflour, 4 tablespoons
- Salt, 1 & *1/2* tablespoons
- Dried basil, *1/2* teaspoon
- Mustard powder, 1 tablespoon
- Turmeric powder, 2 tablespoons
- Keen's Traditional Curry Powder, 2 tablespoons
- Sultanas and/or dates (optional)
- Chilli powder (optional)

METHOD
- Quarter and then finely dice the tomatoes and onions. Peel and core the apples and finely chop them.
- Add the prepared fruit and vegetables to a large pot along with all the other ingredients, and mix. For a bit of variety and depending on taste, you might wish to reduce the amount of sugar and/or replace some of the sugar with sultanas and/or chopped dates. If you would like a bit of extra 'kick' to the relish, you can also add some chilli powder to taste.
- Cook your relish mixture on low heat for 90 minutes. Depending on how plump and juicy the tomatoes were, a little extra cornflour may be

required to achieve the desired final consistency. If you feel additional cornflour is needed, mix it smoothly with water before adding it to the pot and cooking for a further ten minutes.
- Bottle the relish in sterilised jars while it is still hot.
- Serve the relish as accompaniment to any food that takes your fancy. It's great on sandwiches and wraps, and on cheese platters with cheese and biscuits. In fact, my daughter says it's good with ANYTHING and EVERYTHING!

S.   'S' IS FOR 'START RIGHT NOW'

Don't wait, just START RIGHT NOW!

If you wish to be happy, don't think of this only as a far-off state. Embrace the journey to happiness by starting on it right NOW. Happiness is not only a future condition, but needs to be nurtured in the beginning, to exist in the here and now. You create your own happiness, and you need to work on it now.

Three important things to remember:
- Don't put your thoughts on the idea that one day, someone will make you happy.
- Know that you create your own happiness – only you.
- START RIGHT NOW on being happy.

Garden Tip 'S':
- *Let's grow sorrel!*

In the spring I sow sorrel seeds in a small pot, 1 cm deep, and when the seedlings are large enough to handle, I move them to individual pots, keeping them in a warm and bright spot. When planting out into a garden keep them 0.5 cm deep and 30 cm apart. Protect them from pets and weather until they are established. Water them only once or twice a week;

they don't like wet feet. They can be an invasive plant so keeping them in pots is great. When the leaves are about 4 cm long it's time to harvest. The tender leaves are best for eating so harvest from the aerial outer leaves on a 'cut and come again' principle, where you will have a steady supply for the season. If the leaves get too big simply cut them back. Be sure to remove the flowers if you want to keep producing the leaves (but reserve some to let go to seed to be collected for next season).

Besides the leaves of sorrel making a great salad vegetable, sorrel also has medicinal benefits, but DO NOT OVEREAT IT and DO NOT CONSUME THE PLANT OR ITS MEDICINAL DERIVATIVES IN LARGE AMOUNTS. Where carefully prepared and used in appropriate amounts, sorrel can be beneficial for reduction of pain and swelling, and reducing inflammation of the nasal passages and respiratory tract. It can also be good for use against bacterial infections. It is a strong diuretic and has been used against cancers too.

> **WARNING: EATING SORREL SEEDS CAN BE TOXIC.**
> Ingesting too much sorrel can also cause diarrhoea, nausea, increased urination, skin reactions, stomach and digestive issues, eye irritation, eye damage and kidney damage.

Natural Therapy Thought 'S':
- *Sunshine.*

Try to get 20 minutes of sunshine a day, while staying sun-smart, of course! This is necessary for us to produce our own vitamin D. Vitamin D is important for our bones, blood cells and immune system. It also assists us to absorb certain minerals from our diet, including calcium and phosphorus. Sunshine can also boost mood, improve sleep quality, and reduce stress.

Favourite Food Thought 'S':
- *Sauerkraut.*

Sauerkraut is a wonderfully vibrant fermented food with a delicious and deep flavour. And this is just from combining cabbage and salt!

I used to deal a lot with raw and fermented foods when I worked at a health food store, and in conjunction with the Rudolf Steiner School that my daughter attended as a child. I am so pleased to see the recent rise of fermented food in this modern age, with knowledge passed from the old ages!

There are SO many health benefits of fermented food, in a variety of ways. Fermented food improves digestion, aids in lowering the risk of certain diseases (including diabetes and heart disease), and crucially can promote a healthy and diverse microbiome (the collection of organisms living in your gut).

Sauerkraut may seem like something that's too complicated to make at home, but you might be surprised at how easy it can actually be. If you'd like to try making it yourself, here is a favourite sauerkraut recipe from the wonderful Nourished Kitchen website online:
https://nourishedkitchen.com/homemade-sauerkraut/

T.   'T' IS FOR 'THINK FOR YOURSELF'

Your happiness is what you make it, not what others give to you.

You control your own happiness. Like-minded people can join you and work on happiness with you, but your happiness comes from within you – it is your thoughts, your actions, and your beliefs that all combine to create your own happiness.

Three important things to remember:
- Don't be controlled by others.
- Do your best, not what others expect of you.
- Your happiness comes from what you give yourself.

Garden Tip 'T':
- *Turnips.*

The most forgotten vegetable, in my opinion, along with parsnips (oh, and carrots too, actually!).

Dad used to grow turnips and parsnips en masse and share them with the community. And I put turnips and parsnips into most things I make – they are both equally my favourites.

To grow these wonderful root vegetables (including the carrots, too), first sow your seeds directly into little trenches in dampened soil. Cover with more soil and water in immediately. Place a plank of wood over the soil-covered and watered channel. In a few days remove the plank as you will see tiny seedlings.

Parsnips and carrots will grow down while the turnips will become a ball-shape (the turnips should be around the size of golf balls after at least ten weeks or so). Start checking for harvesting opportunities after about eight weeks. If the vegetable is visible from under the dirt (protruding), then it is time to collect it. Rinse and enjoy, or if you are like my daughter, just brush off the soil and eat it right there where you stand!

Natural Therapy Thought 'T':
- *Treat a toothache.*

Chew on cloves or ginger root.

The following may also help: clove oil, tea tree oil, chamomile, willow bark, vitamin A, vitamin C, vitamin E, bromelain, quercetin, silica, magnesium, Bach's Rescue Remedy, and homeopathic calcarea phosphorica (Calc Phos), magnesium phosphate (Mag Phos), and potassium phosphate (Kali Phos).

Favourite Recipe 'T':
- *English tomato and onion pie.*

This delicious savoury pie is a real favourite of my husband, who is also English!

INGREDIENTS
- Sweet onions, 8 cups, thinly sliced
- Tomatoes, medium, 3-4, thinly sliced (plus additional slices, optional)
- Butter, 2 tablespoons
- Bacon strips, 12, cooked and drained
- Soft breadcrumbs, 2 cups
- Cheddar cheese, shredded, 2 cups
- Eggs, 3 large
- Salt, *1/4* teaspoon
- Pepper, *1/8* teaspoon

METHOD
- In a large skillet, sauté the onions in butter until tender.
- Crumble nine of the cooked bacon strips in a bowl.
- Place the breadcrumbs in a greased 9-inch deep-dish pie plate.
- Layer the breadcrumbs with half of the following, in order: tomatoes, onions, crumbled bacon, and cheese. Top with the remaining tomatoes, then the onions, then the crumbled bacon.
- In a bowl, beat together the eggs and salt and pepper.
- Pour the egg liquid over the top of the pie layers. Sprinkle the surface of the pie with the remaining cheese. Top the pie with the three remaining (uncrumbled) bacon strips. Place extra tomato slices around the edge of the pie, if desired.
- Bake the pie at 180 degrees Celsius for 35-40 minutes or until a knife inserted into the centre comes out clean.
- Let the pie stand for ten minutes before cutting and serving.
- Refrigerate any leftovers.

U. 'U' IS FOR 'UNLEASH YOUR ENERGY'

The hard work of happiness can require a lot of energy.

The 'happiness business' doesn't work if you are unwilling to put in the effort. It is hard work, and needs patience, perseverance, and ENERGY. Do what you need to do to create and release your energy needed to work on achieving your happiness. Allow your energy release to release your highest thoughts and actions.

Three important things to remember:
- Life does not do things for you – you do them yourself.
- Let your energy generate what you want to do, and then do it.
- Unleash your highest thoughts.

Garden Tip 'U':
- *Umbelliferae.*

This term refers to a group of plants that have umbrella-like flowers. They are those cooking staples, carrot and celery and parsley. I consider them to be garden essentials! Dad grew all of these, of course, including the many kinds of parsley (the umbrella-head flowers form when it goes to seed). Parsley is actually my favourite herb, and I eat it every day.

Natural Therapy Thought 'U':
- *Unani therapy.*

Much like the Indian ayurvedic medicine that I mentioned earlier in this chapter (see section 'O'), Unani is a very old system of medicine and therapy, although the principles of the two methods differ somewhat. Unani medicine was developed in the Middle East and is based on the teachings of the ancient Greeks Hippocrates and Galen. It is a philosophy of balancing the external elements and body humours, chiefly by way of physical therapy, diet, and natural medicines. It is used to treat a variety of ailments and conditions, with particularly promising results being reported through its use in treating autoimmune disorders of the skin. Certainly my daughter has had great outcomes for those patients she treats for these issues by applying Unani therapies in her clinic.

Favourite Food Thought 'U':
- *Unagi.*

Unagi are Japanese sushi rolls, and they are one of my favourite things. Making your own is so easy and you can put in whatever you want, and/or omit what you are allergic to (or just what doesn't meet your own food preferences).

My daughter makes hers in an egg carton to save herself the rolling process. She first lines the carton with cling-wrap, then places a piece of salmon in the bottom of each little carton cup-hole (where the eggs had originally rested). She then layers in sliced avocado, a square of sea-vegetable wrap, some cucumber, some pre-prepared sushi rice, and her chosen sauce. She covers the layered cup-holes with more cling-wrap and squishes each sushi combo down, then leaves the whole thing in the fridge overnight. The next day she turns the unagi out into their individual portions to serve – so easy to eat!

V.   'V' IS FOR 'VALUE WHAT YOU HAVE'

Be grateful for the happiness you have.

It is important to appreciate and be grateful for the happiness you already have, even when you are working on improving it. Even especially when you are working on improving it, because the existing happiness will also encourage you to keep on striving for more. Give thanks and be grateful also for your own positivity and motivation, and know that because of them you can attract others who are positive too. You can all progress on the happiness journey together!

Three important things to remember:
- Be grateful that you have the ability to have what you want.
- You have positivity – use it.
- If you want happiness, go for it!

Garden Tip 'V':
- *The value of home-grown vegetables.*

This is so simple.
From the mouth of Mother: "It tastes REAL when you grow it yourself. There is just no flavour in the bought ones."
I rest my case.

Natural Therapy Thought 'V':
- *Varicose vein treatment.*

Calendula – used topically, and as a tea. Verbena tea and rosehip tea. Equisetum (horsetail herb), vitamin B, vitamin C, vitamin E. Buckwheat, calcium, silica. Homeopathic calcarea carbonica. Arnica is great for rapid healing, and pulsatilla is also good for reducing the swelling of varicose veins.

Favourite Recipe 'V':
- *Vanilla muffins.*

Vanilla beans are a culinary blessing, and preparing a vanilla bean to use in cooking is easy.

For most recipes, use a sharp knife to slice the bean in half lengthways while leaving the underside intact. Then scrape the seeds out and incorporate them into the dish's other ingredients according to the specific recipe. The outer pod can also be used to infuse the vanilla flavour into milk, cream or sugar.

Most often, vanilla beans are processed commercially into vanilla extract, a common ingredient in baked goods and other sweet food recipes. Don't drink this, but DO smell its wonderful smell! It will make you happy, possibly more than you are aware of (please make sure you check out section 'X' – yes, 'X' – in this chapter too, for how vanilla is also good for physical and mental health).

I have a lovely vanilla muffin recipe to share here – a deceptively simple combination of flour, butter, sugar, eggs, and a generous amount of vanilla extract or paste. You might not think much of this recipe at first glance, but it is easy to make and the results are tender, moist, and lightly sweet muffins that need little to no embellishment. However, if you would like to fancy them up a little for serving, they could be accompanied by raspberry or strawberry preserves, marmalade, or your favourite jam. For extra fanciness and sweetness you could also drizzle the cooled muffins with a tablespoon of vanilla glaze. The muffins make a simple delicious breakfast, are the perfect partner for a cup of coffee or tea, and can be a wonderful dessert in their dressed-up variations.

INGREDIENTS
- All-purpose flour, 4 cups (about 480 g)
- Granulated sugar, 2 cups
- Baking powder, 1 tablespoon plus 2 teaspoons
- Salt, *3/4* teaspoon
- Milk, 2 cups
- Butter, *1/2* cup, melted
- Eggs, 2 large
- Vanilla extract, 1 tablespoon (or *1/4* teaspoon vanilla bean paste)

METHOD
- Preheat the oven to 200 degrees Celsius.
- Grease 24 cups of a muffin tray or line them with paper.
- In a large bowl, combine the flour, sugar, baking powder, and salt. Stir to mix thoroughly.
- In a medium bowl, whisk together the milk, butter, eggs, and vanilla extract/paste until combined.
- Pour the wet mixture into the dry ingredients and use a spoon to mix thoroughly.
- Spoon the batter into the prepared muffin-tray cups.
- Bake in the preheated oven for about 15-20 minutes. Note that a dark

tray will take less time than a light-coloured tray. The muffins are done when a toothpick or cake-tester comes out clean when inserted into the middle of a muffin.
- Remove the muffins from the tray and cool them on a rack.
- Serve and enjoy!

W.   'W' IS FOR 'WALK EVERY DAY'

Walking is wonderful.

Wherever physically possible, go for a walk, daily if you can. Walking aids your physical body and it nourishes your mental body too. The exercise assists the muscles while the 'time to think' allows you to work on yourself. Walking with friends and animals also adds to the happiness of walking.

Three important things to remember:
- Walking exercises the body and the mind.
- Walk near nature to create natural happiness.
- Walk with a friend or an animal for extra happiness.

Garden Tip 'W':
- *Walk around the garden.*

This is an activity, but it's also a destination.
I have many fond recollections of visiting with my parents and the first thing we would do would be to walk around the garden. It was a way of saying hello, and connecting, too. We would spend at least 45 minutes out front in the 'blooms' garden with Mother, then at least the same time out back with Dad in the 'edibles' area, his beloved vegetable garden. Walk, walk, walk…even with Mother's bunion feet and aching knees, and Dad with his various body ailments, we all walked for interest, health, and communication. The same conversations would not have been had around

a kitchen table, nor would they have flowed indoors as they did outdoors. 'Garden time' runs away from you, and then the day seems to vanish quickly. Darkness falls. "Oh, is it that time already?" we would say. Such magical memories.

Natural Therapy Thought 'W':
- *Water.*

The hero of nature. Drink it, bathe in it, soak in it, play in it… And what about the magic of splashing in puddles, or standing in the pouring rain? Just ask little kids!

Water is the liquid of life, and it's your health's best friend.

Favourite Recipe 'W':
- *Walnut and feta hot-roasted beetroot.*

I have been a massive fan of walnuts over the years. I pop them in and on desserts, cakes, loaves, crumbles, and tarts. I put them in my overnight oats, and include them in my ground nut and seed mix that I sprinkle on my cereal. I love them in salads! They are such a great source of alpha-linolenic acid, an omega-3 fatty acid, which can reduce inflammation and help address heart disease too.

Here is a casual and simple recipe for walnut and feta hot-roasted beetroot.

INGREDIENTS

(Determine your own companion ingredient proportions by personal taste and with reference to your starting beet quantity.)
- Fresh beetroots with their tops on, 4
- Rocket
- Feta cheese chunks
- Olive oil
- Leeks and/or onions, chopped finely
- Chives to taste, chopped finely
- Basil to taste, either dried or fresh
- Walnuts, roasted

- Salt
- Pepper

METHOD
- Preheat the oven to 200 degrees Celsius.
- Wash and peel the beetroots and cut them into chunks. Place them on a baking tray, drizzle with oil and bake until soft to preference. Add salt and pepper to taste.
- In a bowl, combine all other ingredients and then mix with the soft beetroots, adjusting seasoning further to taste as required. Place the mixture in a baking dish and bake in the oven for a further 15 minutes.
- Sprinkle with extra feta and walnuts and serve hot.

X.   'X' IS FOR 'X-PECT ONLY THE BEST'

Your expectation of the best is a big plus.

You deserve the best, so why not X-PECT it? Work towards expecting and receiving the best and the most that you can get, to assist with achieving your happiness.

Three important things to remember:
- Expectation is very powerful.
- Expect only the best of what you want.
- If you expect only a little, you will receive only a little – expect more to get more!

Garden Tip 'X':
- *X-tra garden guests!*

One day my brother and his older daughter, my oldest niece, were walking around inspecting their family's garden (yes, my brother and sister-in-law were also great gardeners, and Mother and I would often help out with their latest garden work, whenever we visited them). The family dog, a beautiful blue heeler and border collie cross named Tess, was also there, running around and chewing the air enthusiastically near the flowering bushes. My brother remarked, "Silly dog, I don't know how she doesn't get stung, snapping at the bees like that." My niece took a closer look, and replied, "Those aren't bees, those are hoverflies – no stings there!" Well, my brother gained a lot of respect for the insect-distinguishing talents of dogs that day! Dear Tess has since passed on, but I like to think that my brother remembers her fondly whenever he sees the bees (or are they hoverflies?) in his garden now.

This story illustrates that the nature we can appreciate in gardens is not limited to plants – there are lots of little animals around, too. Some of them are unwelcome (see section 'K' in this chapter for how you might deal with those!) but some of them are truly desirable 'guests'. Not least, of course, our wonderful pollinator friends, the bees. But also ladybirds, because the adults and the larvae both eat aphid pests. Lacewings and praying mantises and spiders likewise can assist with getting rid of pests (and please do look up what ladybird and lacewing larvae look like, not only to make sure you recognise and let them stay in your garden, but because they are just amazing-looking things). Even simple animals such as springtails and earthworms are good for the soil. Your welcomed garden friends will add to the happiness you find in your garden, and in simply enjoying the little creatures for their own sakes, too.

Natural Therapy Thought 'X':
- *X-tra vanilla!*

Besides making for delightfully delicious muffins (see the 'V' section of this chapter), you should know that vanilla has more to offer than just the flavouring of food.

Did you know that medicinally, vanilla has been used in the treatment of sickle cell anaemia? Vanilla possesses chemoreactive properties, which help to prevent cellular degradation such as that found in sickle cell anaemia.

Vanilla also is great for relieving anxiety. In concentrated, medicinal forms, the main compounds of vanilla have been shown to affect the central nervous system, stimulating production of the 'happy hormone' serotonin and helping to reduce anxiety and depression. It's no wonder we like to cook with it!

Favourite Recipe 'X':
- *X-tra pie (Scottish treacle tart)!*

I had two lovely candidate recipes for 'T'. I ended up putting a savoury English tomato and onion pie in that section.

The other 'T' candidate I had was Scottish treacle tart, which could be considered a sweet pie! I thought it would be a real shame to leave its recipe out of this book just because its letter was already used. Also it was Dad's favourite treat.

So let's not say no to extra 'pie'!

Treacle tart is a traditional British dessert that's rich and comforting. It is best served with a splash of cream.

INGREDIENTS
- Shortcrust pastry, 225 g
- Butter, 60 g
- Golden syrup, 400 g
- Treacle, 35 g
- Double cream, 2 tablespoons
- Egg, 1 whole (reserve a little for the egg wash for the pastry)
- Egg, 1 yolk only
- Lemon juice, 1 tablespoon
- Porridge oats, 140 g

METHOD
- Preheat the oven to 180 degrees Celsius.
- Grease a pie dish and then lay the pastry into the bottom of the dish. Prick the pastry all over with a fork then lay a sheet of foil over it. Fill the base with baking beans.
- Blind-bake the shell in the oven for 15 minutes. Remove the baking beans and foil. Brush the pastry base with egg wash or milk, then bake for

another five minutes until golden.
- Melt the butter in a pan over medium heat. Watch it carefully as it can burn quickly, but it's all right if it goes a little brown, as that just adds a nutty flavour to the treacle mixture.
- Add the golden syrup and the treacle to the melted butter. Heat and stir.
- Take the mixture off the heat and mix in the cream.
- Beat in the whole egg, yolk, and lemon juice.
- Sprinkle the porridge oats evenly over the pastry crust base.
- Pour the treacle filling over the porridge oats, making sure there are no dry patches.
- Bake in the oven for 20 minutes, then turn the oven down to 140 degrees Celsius and bake for another 15 minutes.
- Allow to cool and then serve with cream.

Y. 'Y' IS FOR 'YOU ARE IMPORTANT'

You are important, for there is only one you.

You are unique and important. Value yourself and work on your self-esteem – BELIEVE that you are important. Self-confidence and a sense of your own importance in the world will give you more courage to improve yourself and your happiness. Never stop working on yourself and your happiness, and never stop believing in yourself and your right to happiness.

Three important things to remember:
- You cannot be happy without self-value.
- If your self-esteem is low, work on it, and raise it up.
- Apply your belief in yourself to grow your happiness.

Garden Tip 'Y':
- *Yellow archangel.*

This is a member of the mint family. It has beautiful bright-yellow flowers and silver-streaked leaves, and loves to form a thick carpet of plants in the shade of trees. In fact, yellow archangel grows so well that it can easily spread beyond your intentions, and because of this it is treated as an invasive weed in some places. It is a perfect example to show that when you create a garden, you also need to be in control of it.

Natural Therapy Thought 'Y':
- *Yoga.*

It is important to move your body, and to move it in the right way for your own health and happiness requirements. I have been a practitioner of yoga for most of my life; it is gentle and spiritual and so very effective for me. There are many variations and many teachers, whether they be Indian gurus or Hollywood actresses (I practised Raquel Welch's methods for years). These days the internet makes it very easy to find and follow those yoga methods that will resonate specifically with you – what a great meeting of ancient wisdom and modern technology.

Favourite Recipe 'Y':
- *Yummiest coconut loaf cake.*

This is also one of my daughter's recipes. It makes me so happy to share her wonderful baking creations with you, and I know that she is equally as delighted to share. She and I are both all about wellness and happiness, and this lovely cake will create a lot of both in those who make and consume it.

INGREDIENTS
- Desiccated coconut, 1 cup
- Shredded coconut, 1 cup, plus a little extra for decoration (optional)
- Coconut oil (melted), 1 cup, plus a little extra for drizzling (optional)
- Fine sugar, *1/2* cup
- Eggs, 3

- Vanilla essence, 2 teaspoons
- Self-raising flour (or gluten-free flour alternative), *1/2* cup
- Baking powder, 1 teaspoon
- Maple syrup, for drizzling (optional)

METHOD
- Mix the sugar, cup of coconut oil, eggs and vanilla essence in a bowl.
- Add the baking powder and flour and mix.
- Add the desiccated coconut and the cup of shredded coconut and mix.
- Pour the mixture into a lined loaf tin.
- Bake at 180 degrees Celsius for 30 minutes or until a skewer comes out clean.
- If desired, and while the cake is still warm, drizzle over a mixture of the maple syrup and the additional coconut oil (this makes the cake extra-moist) and decorate the top with a little more shredded coconut.

Z.   'Z' IS FOR 'ZILCH'

Whatever you put into life is what you get back.

If you put in zilch effort, you get zilch results! In order to succeed you need to apply yourself. If you work positively, putting in lots of effort, you will achieve your goals and desires. Work on your happiness with positivity, and your happiness will flow.

Three important things to remember:
- Results do not come without effort.
- Work hard towards positive results and you will succeed.
- Work on THINKING happy, DOING happy, and BEING happy!

Garden Tip 'Z':
- *Zingiber officinale.*

This is the scientific name for common ginger. Easy to grow in either a garden bed or as a pot-plant, its root is great for use in cooking and it is magic medicinally. And its flowers! Many people are much less familiar with its beautiful flowers, but I absolutely love them and they do very well as cut blooms in a vase.

Natural Therapy Thought 'Z':
- *Zingiber officinale.*

No, it's not déjà vu. As mentioned above, ginger is medicinally MAGIC; I would need a whole extra chapter to list all of its uses and benefits! Most people already know that it is great as an anti-nausea remedy (very useful against seasickness). Ginger has strong antioxidant properties and may help manage arthritis. Chewing fresh ginger is also great for the gut, cutting down on gas and bloating, and alleviating constipation. If you don't want to chew it, the easiest way to consume it is to make ginger tea – simply place fresh ginger slices in a mug and add hot water!

> **WARNING: GINGER MAY NOT BE FOR EVERYONE.**
> Some people may be more sensitive to the effects of ginger, especially if those people have or are being treated/medicated for certain conditions. Please consult with your own doctor before consuming ginger or ginger supplements, particularly if you are pregnant or breastfeeding, have or are being treated for coronary heart/artery disease, or are diabetic and taking insulin.

Favourite Recipe 'Z':
- *Zucchini soup.*

Once when I was visiting with my oldest niece, she made a delicious zucchini soup for our lunch. Later when I asked her for the recipe she said she didn't really have one. She said she was a 'taste-as-you-go' kind of cook, at least where soup was concerned! She has finally written down the basics of the recipe here, but wants everyone to remember this advice: "Don't sweat the details – just make it your own!"

INGREDIENTS
- Green zucchini, 3-5
- Brown onion, 1 (or equivalent onion powder)
- White potato, 1
- Chicken-flavoured stock cubes/powder and/or liquid chicken-flavoured stock, equivalent to at least one litre
- Parsley, fresh or dried, equivalent to about *1/2* teaspoon dried
- Butter, 2 tablespoons (or equivalent oil)
- Water
- Milk, about *1/2* cup (optional)
- Salt
- Pepper

METHOD
- Wash the zucchini and remove and discard the very ends. Do not peel. Cut the zucchini roughly into half-circle slices.
- If you are using a fresh onion, peel and chop it.
- Wash and peel the potato and chop it into rough smaller chunks.
- Add the butter (or oil) to a large saucepan (with plenty of room for stirring based on the vegetable quantity you have prepared) and melt it over medium heat.
- Add the zucchini to the saucepan and stir constantly over the heat as the zucchini begins to cook, but don't let it or the pot interior get brown. This part is important to get the most vibrant green possible from the zucchini to impart to the soup. When the zucchini skin has turned a brighter green and the flesh is just starting to soften, go to the next step.

- Add the potato, onion, parsley, and stock cubes/powder/liquid. Add any water needed to make up at least one litre of soup, and in any case covering above the vegetables by at least two centimetres. Place a lid on the saucepan, bring the mixture to the boil, then slow-boil or simmer until the vegetables are soft. (Note: Using only a vegetable-based 'chicken' stock such as from Massel will make the soup vegetarian. To make it vegan, additionally substitute out the butter for oil and leave out the milk. And provided that your stock and seasonings are wheat-free, the soup will also be gluten free.)
- Once the vegetables are soft, turn off the heat, and if necessary, remove the saucepan to a suitable alternative heat-proof surface. Add the milk (if using). Blend the soup until it is smooth and consistent, using a stick blender. (If you don't have a stick blender, a potato masher can be used but the soup will just have a bit more texture.)
- Add salt and pepper to taste, and if necessary adjust the thickness and taste of the soup as desired via more water/milk/stock/whatever – make it your own!
- Return the soup to low heat for long enough to make sure it is the preferred temperature for serving (avoid boiling it if it now contains milk).
- Serve the soup on its own, or it is also nice garnished with shredded cheddar cheese and/or accompanied by some fresh bread and butter.

And there it is – the end of my Happy Alphabet. YOU NOW HAVE HAPPINESS! So, I repeat:

The secret to happiness is the choice to be a happy person.

3. Healing Myself for Happiness.

This is just a little chapter of a few of the things that I have done and continue to do to look after my physical and mental health, to promote my happiness through healing myself.

You may find something here that works for you, too!

1.   HOMEOPATHY

I believe there is a place for both conventional medicine and homeopathy in a person's wellness and happiness journey, should the person wish it. For me, homeopathy has saved my life! The key is for each individual to find what suits their particular needs, wants and health considerations.

I have been plagued with headaches all my life. Long ago it was suggested to me to try herbal teas, so I did. Lavender and peppermint have been successful in combatting headaches in others, but unfortunately for me, I was allergic to those particular teas and to many others besides! Happily, one I could tolerate was chamomile. I have now been drinking chamomile flower tea for over 60 years as a wonderfully refreshing way to keep my headaches at bay.

If you wish to explore what homeopathy might be able to do for you and your health and happiness, I encourage you to check out the many books and articles online and in physical print. I would also suggest having a discussion with or an assessment by a homeopathic professional (I happen to know a very good one called Dr. Dee – see her contact details on page 91 of this book!) to work out your customised homeopathic program.

2.   HEAT

Heat has been a saving grace in my life. Not only does it feel cosy and like a mother's warm hug, but it brings blood to your body's surface, reduces stiffness and muscle spasms, and addresses pain. So consider a little warming for health and happiness – heat applications, heat compresses, warm drinks, warm baths, warm coverings, basking in the sun...

Back in the 1980s, a few times every year I would attend a health retreat in the Dandenong Ranges on the outskirts of Melbourne, Victoria. One of the highlights for me was the hot thermal mineral pools. I was transported to a different time, space and galaxy with each blissful thermal experience. For me it was the combination of the heat, the minerals and the 'knowing' this was good for me. There was also an icy plunge pool that we were encouraged to dunk in after a certain time interval, and then return to the thermal bliss. Today, taking a hot-water bottle to bed with me is just as blissful. As I lie there, I remember all the good those thermal experiences did for me, and I imagine and feel it in the present, too. There is a warm spa here where we live now but I have not been there yet. The heat of the sunshine is also blissful and medicinal to sit in daily – interestingly, I don't go so well in the cold!

The heat is wonderful and offers peace and tranquillity along with its healing powers.

I find it very beneficial, once my back has had a heat application, to do one of my favourite little exercises – 'Feet Up The Wall'. Just sit on the floor near the wall, facing the wall. Tuck your knees up to your chest and move and support yourself until your back is lying flat on the floor, arms out by your sides, and your legs are up the wall, straight, so that you are looking up at your feet. This has helped to relieve my back tension and headaches, and assisted to prevent protruding veins and normalise my blood pressure. Other reported benefits of this simple technique are asthma relief, toning of the glandular system, thyroid function improvement, insomnia relief, and assistance with easing depression. By no means is this medical advice, but I have found this exercise has been very useful for me (and for others to whom I have recommended it) over the past 60 years.

3. CHANGE YOUR BREATH AND FEEL BETTER

One day, I found an article in a wellbeing magazine that I thought was so interesting I just had to show it first to my daughter, then to a dear friend of mine, and then to an old colleague. It was all about how controlling your breathing could help the health of both your body and mind.

I nearly fell off my seat when I read the article, because I have been practising various breathing techniques for many years (since I was a ballroom dancer-turned-teacher in the 1970s) and I was so excited to see an article by medical professionals recognising the benefits of breathing exercises.

You may think that breathing just happens and that's all there is to it, but no, good breathing is an art form. A relaxed human adult naturally takes about 840 breaths per hour, without giving it much or any thought. So could you imagine the potential difference to a person's wellness and happiness if even a few of those breaths were taken with the specific purpose and intention to enhance their health? It's because someone's oxygen levels not only dictate their physical performance capabilities, but can have a profound impact on their stress levels, mind and mental health, and HAPPINESS.

A little research will show that many breathing techniques are available for you to try to see what might work for you. Below are four that I have found useful for myself for maintaining and enhancing my own health and happiness.

Cupped Hand Breath
Do this when you feel you have been burning the candle at both ends.
    (a) Sit quietly.
    (b) Cup your hands and place them over your eyes.
    (c) Hold your hands over your eyes for 10 seconds while taking a breath in and out.
    (d) Gently remove your hands and look at your palms.
    (e) Repeat from step (b).
    (f) Do 10 rounds in total, and enjoy the feeling of peacefulness.

Sun Breath (Alternate Nostril Breathing)
Do this when you want to increase your energy and vitality, as this will warm the body and allow you to become more alert.
    (a) In a seated position, place your right hand on your right knee.
    (b) Breathe out completely.
    (c) Use your left thumb to block off your left nostril.
    (d) Take a full deep breath through your right nostril, hold, and then gently close your right nostril with your left ring finger.
    (e) Move your left thumb to unblock your left nostril, and breathe out completely through your left nostril.

(f) Breathe in through your left nostril, hold, and then gently close your left nostril again with your left thumb.
(g) Move your left ring finger to unblock your right nostril.
(h) Breathe out through your right nostril, to complete round one.
(i) Start the process again from step (d).
(j) Repeat slowly for 10 rounds in total.

Golden Thread Breath
Do this when you are feeling stressed and overwhelmed.
(a) Sit comfortably.
(b) Slowly breathe in and out – in through your nose, and out through gently parted lips.
(c) On each out-breath, imagine a fine golden thread being spun like fairy floss (AKA candy floss, AKA cotton candy) out of your mouth, and getting longer and going further and further away from you as each breath you exhale deepens.
(d) On each in-breath, imagine that your energy levels are being replenished with a golden mist, that then increases the material for the golden thread as each breath you inhale deepens too.
(e) Be aware that all of your 'cloudy clutter' is being removed and replaced with a vibrant golden power to fuel you.

Feather Breath
Do this when you are hot and bothered and need to slow down your heart rate.
(a) Sit comfortably and imagine you are holding a soft fluffy feather in your fingertips, in front of your face.
(b) Slowly breathe in and out through your gently parted lips, blowing your imaginary feather so that you can 'see' its wispy edges moving, and feel the coolness of your breath blowing over your fingers.

4. THREE-MINUTE NECK AND SHOULDER STRETCH

I have done many health courses in my life, and while I can't remember which one taught me this kind of stretch, I just want to share the technique with the world. I have found that it is most effective when done while in the shower under the hot water, or in a warm bath, or after applying a hot compress.

This simple exercise has saved me from pain and tension for more than 50 years.

THE STRETCHING, STEP-BY-STEP
- (a) Start by sitting or standing up and looking straight ahead.
- (b) Inhale and count to 5 while turning your head to the right, to look across your right shoulder.
- (c) Hold your position and count to 5 while you exhale.
- (d) Return your head to the front, and repeat three times.
- (e) Once you have completed the three to-the-right motions and your head is back facing forward, you will be doing the same motions but to the left instead.
- (f) Inhale and count to 5 while turning your head to the left, to look across your left shoulder.
- (g) Hold your position and count to 5 while you exhale.
- (h) Return your head to the front, and repeat three times.
- (i) Once you have completed the three to-the-left motions, you will be facing forward again.
- (j) Keep looking straight ahead and breathe normally while you tilt your right ear to your right shoulder (do NOT bring your shoulder up to your ear) and hold for 10 seconds, then return your head to upright.
- (k) Repeat the same movement and count for the left side, remembering to keep looking straight ahead and breathe normally.

(l) Now tilt your head forward, chin to chest, and hold for 10 seconds.
(m) Finally, roll your SHOULDERS up, back and down 10 times SLOWLY AT A SNAIL'S PACE.
(n) Remember not to hold your breath while doing the stretches, and ensure not to bounce or make jarring movements which may risk you hurting yourself.
(o) If you have the time and are able to physically do it, I have found that lying on my back on the floor, knees bent and no pillow, has also been beneficial for me after I have completed the stretching technique first.

5. REFLEXOLOGY

THERE IS HELP AND HAPPINESS AFOOT!

For the pure interest of treating myself and my family, reflexology has featured in my life for over 60 years. You may have heard of it before and may even know more about it than you think. I'm not going to explain every single in and out of reflexology here, or how to do it (there are plenty of online resources for that), but I am going to say that as a self-care item and a promoter of happiness, I 100% LOVE reflexology, both giving and receiving.

Reflexology is a form of holistic therapy applied to the hands, the feet and the ears. All parts of the whole body, including internal organs, are mapped out in grids on the hands/feet/ears, and then finger pressure is applied to specific points in the grids. This hands/feet/ears connection to the body organs offers energetic lymph and hormone control, for a large range of health benefits. For me, not only does it have instant results, but long-lasting results too. My daughter practises reflexology professionally in her clinic, and has assisted many people over the years with this gentle therapy. She even has a very old reflexology chart of mine from the 1970s displayed on a wall in her clinic. This makes me happy!

I have lived all my life with different healing modalities, and reflexology has to be one of my very favourites. I know my daughter massages her feet with essential oils nightly before bed, as do I, and so did Mother before me – we all benefited and continue to benefit from this ancient wisdom.

And who doesn't love a foot rub?

6. TAPPING

Tapping is a method of dealing with pain, and it is a wonderful and very underutilised self-healing skill, in my opinion. Those with whom I have shared it over the years have also found it very beneficial. I consider its use to be an integral part of my happiness, and of my choosing to be happy about my life. For me, sometimes the relief is instant.

The method is very straightforward – you simply use the first three fingers of your right hand to tap gently several times on sequential 'tapping points' on your face and chest, while vocalising your pain.

Following are the steps of how you would undertake a tapping if, for example, you had pain in your left foot. A diagram is included to illustrate the 16 tapping points of the head and face (a 17th and final point is below your ribs).

> **(1)** Tap the top of your head and say the vocalisation, "I have pain **in my left foot**, but I'm okay."

(2) Tap the centre of your forehead and say, "I have pain **in my left foot**, but I'm okay."

(3) Tap between your eyebrows, repeating the vocalisation as you tap the new point.

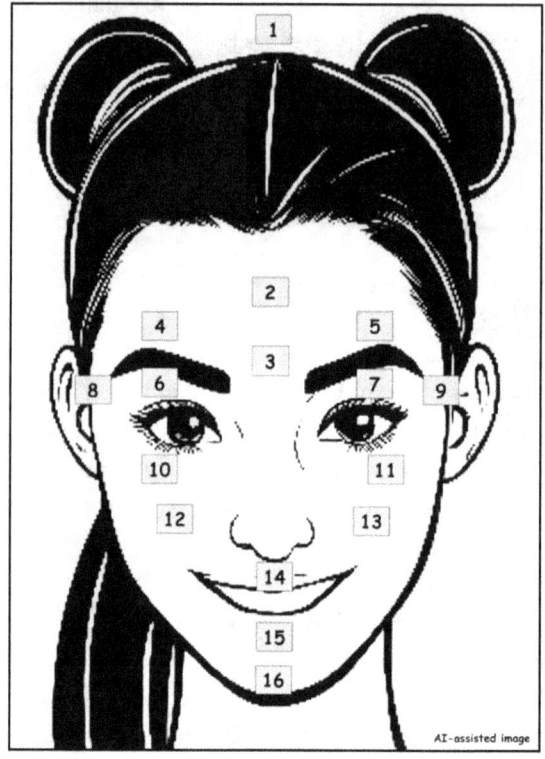

(4) (5) Tap above each eyebrow as indicated, and vocalise as you tap each new point.

(6) (7) Below each eyebrow – tap and vocalise.

(8) (9) On each temple – tap and vocalise.

(10) (11) Below each eye – tap and vocalise.

(12) (13) On each cheek – tap and vocalise.

(14) Above the mouth – tap and vocalise.

(15) Below the mouth – tap and vocalise.
(16) On the chin – tap and vocalise.
(17) Centrally below the ribs – tap and vocalise one final time.

To use this technique to address any type of pain, simply substitute out the actual location of your pain where the above steps have '**in my left foot**'. If you have pain in multiple locations, DON'T change up the pain locations as you tap. Instead, do the tapping technique through all 17 points while vocalising ONE location of pain, then go through a new sequence of all 17 tapping points while vocalising the SECOND location of pain, and so on.

7. ABSENT (DISTANT) HEALING

Absent (distant) healing is used by and for those who are unable to visit a healer in person. I love that there is this ability for people to access the energy and intention of others, from wherever one person is to wherever another is, without the need for physical contact. The healing energy is available to everyone because it extends throughout the world, and transcends time and space.

As a focus for the healing process, I use the plant kingdom. I have my special plant as my focal point. If you try this technique, you should choose a plant especially for yourself. I don't just mean a species of plant – I mean a specific individual plant.

My focus plant even has a name – 'I AM'. She is a bonsai Norfolk pine and she is at least 50 years old.

In using a special focal plant, we aid the healing process as we are tapping into the plant kingdom's vast natural reservoir of pure energy. From all of this you would understand the importance of the feelings you have towards your plant.

Technique:
- Sit quietly with your plant for around 10 minutes each day, at these times.
    - 6.00 am
    - 8.00 am
    - 4.00 pm
    - 6.00 pm
- Concentrate on your plant and imagine being well in yourself.
- Do NOT think about your sickness/disease or troubles.
- Think only of WELLNESS and HAPPINESS. Being whole and well. Picture yourself in vibrant health – the best health imaginable.

Absent healing takes place every day all over the world, so trust that you will get the help needed and that you will give the help needed by others elsewhere. The power is there, always. ALWAYS and INFINITELY.

8. CRYSTAL CLEAR 'COSMIC' HAPPINESS

The eerie screeching was piercing as we entered through the front door. We all looked at each other and the lady behind me tripped over the top step and nearly bowled us all over. The Crystal Healing Retreat was off to a bang of a start!

The screech sounded again. "Oh, isn't she amazing, our alarm?" laughed the retreat's host, Soozi Holbeche, an internationally renowned teacher and practitioner of crystal healing therapy, as she pointed at a large and elaborate birdcage. "She loves hosting our workshops!"

A galah, one of the smaller Australian cockatoos, with beautiful grey-and-pink colouring, sat in the cage flapping her wings and rejoicing at the flow of visitors. We all laughed then, and my young daughter was fascinated. As we approached the cage, the much-loved rescue bird started a dance that Soozi stated she had never seen the galah do before – it wasn't a panic-type dance, but something that almost seemed choreographed. "She does love you, too," Soozi said to my enraptured 12-year-old.

It wasn't even an hour later that Soozi took my arm and said, "We don't usually allow children at my events, but she is an honour to have here, and she is a true healer, Marie!" Soozi allowed my daughter to choose a crystal of her own from the large collection on site that day, and then proceeded to allow her to take charge of the group to share an experience with the room.

"I chose this crystal as I feel it's the most 'breezy'," my daughter said. "I feel the most cool mist coming from it, and if you look into it you can see a pyramid inside it, and wings." She then described her 'electrical' experience: "You see, if you hold it calmly you will see little sparks coming from my fingers, and see them moving around the crystal…"

My 12-year-old daughter had the room ENTHRALLED. I darted a questioning look at Soozi, because a child was taking over her workshop – Soozi simply nodded back to me. My daughter then instructed for the lights to be turned off, and we ALL then witnessed the electrical spark – as did the galah, whose name I now recall (fittingly) was 'Cosmos'. The whole room gasped, including myself and Soozi, and Cosmos danced and danced her choreographed routine. "Ahhh…" Soozi let out a sigh of recognition, "now, THAT is the healing power. If nothing else today, learn how to work with that!"

How amazing, that we can all learn from each other – no matter what the skillset, age or courses taken. We can all work with what we have. It doesn't have to be fancy – the crystal my daughter had chosen was a pink quartz, small and specific. The choices before her that day were vast, including large and elaborate and very expensive crystals and pieces, but she not only chose a little one, but an unassuming one, too. Don't underestimate the innate power within you, no matter how small you may think it could be – it's your spark, your electricity, your happiness.

(Following that retreat, Soozi invited us back for a private session, and she and I had a great chat...while my daughter happily spent her time beside the birdcage, communing with the Cosmos!)

9. HEALTH AND HAPPINESS WITH OTHERS

I have stated repeatedly in this book that happiness is something you give to yourself, rather than something that is bestowed upon you by other people. However, that does not mean that other people don't or can't contribute to the happiness you make for yourself! I have also said that to build your happiness, you need to find joy. One of the most beautiful and powerful sources of joy can be the healthy connections you make to and with family and friends (and even strangers, in some cases).

I have been, and continue to be, so blessed in the family I was given and the friends I have chosen in my life. Every interaction with them that brings me joy builds not only my own happiness but theirs as well. If I do something that makes them happy, that makes me happy. And knowing that they are happy (for whatever reason – I don't have to have been the reason) also makes me happy. It's a win-win situation!

The happiness we give, receive and make in our interactions with others is in itself a great contributor to physical and mental health – a self-propagating cycle of happiness for healing, and healing for happiness.

So take joy in your loved ones, whether it's by having an outing with them doing something grand and exciting, or by simply accessing a favourite memory to lift your spirits on a rainy day. Or anything in between!

It makes me happy to pay tribute here to one of the dearest friends I had in my life, who has been gone for 20 years now. Ena Lemmon, or 'Lemmy' as we called her, was my 'bestie' for so many years. If I think of her I smile, and there it is – a little sprinkle of happiness. Here is an excerpt of a poem that she wrote in the late 1960s (there are many verses – I'm including just the first and last), after she visited and fell in love with the Indian city of Pune (at that time, spelled as 'Poona' in English). Lemmy was a great traveller, and a very spiritual person, too. Her joy and spirit shine out of her words below as she reflects on a day in Poona, and I remember her so fondly whenever I read them.

References explained:
- A 'bund' is an embankment for controlling the flow of water.
- 'Baba Jan' refers to the Afghani/Indian guru, Hazrat Babajan (AKA Hazrat Babajaan, ?-1931). She lived in Pune for the last 25 years of her long life.
- 'Baba Meher' refers to the Indian spiritualist, Meher Baba (1894-1969). He was born in Pune and was a disciple of Baba Jan.

THE MANGO TREE – POONA

Morning bright with sun at the bund in Poona beside the old mango tree.
A sacred spot as Baba Jan and later Meher Baba rested there.
Earlier on, Meher Baba rowed on the broad, slow river.
Today, a flock of birds, brown and white in the distance, skim the water cutting the air like a giant scythe.
On the opposite hill a palace stands majestically, minaret golden against the Indian blue sky.
Below, women busily wash in the river.

Brilliant saris spread in a patchwork along the bank.

Working quietly at his studies, an Indian schoolboy sits near, shyly he interrupts to say that the man beside him is asking if I want someone to do my garden and water my plants.

Well, Australia is my home and it's a bit far to carry the watering can.

Such things happen in India!

* —— *

Now the soft gold sky is reflected in the pearly shimmering river. Moving upstream a rowing boat gently divides the limpid water – ripples of light fan outwards from its path.

A golden peaceful calm wraps the entire evening, as people begin to return homewards.

With its sacred memories the old mango tree stands silent and alone.

Slowly I gather myself together and walk back to my nearby hotel.

This, too, is incredible India!

10.   HOUSESITTING AND WRITING: WORK AND PLAY

With many thanks to my daughter, I can't express how wonderful it is to be having my writings published here for the world to see. Creating this book has been a joy to me, and that makes me happy!

Years ago a great and longtime friend of mine, Ron Pickett, collected some of my thoughts and stories into another happy little booklet that he privately published for my family and close friends. We called the booklet **Marie's Work and Play**, and Ron kindly even wrote a foreword for it. Ron wrote that I was a dear, dear friend (we had attended primary school together in the Victorian country town of Wandong), and he said of me: "During her remarkable life she has shown a flair for the imaginative and creative but has generally been hiding her light under a bushel; here we can see in literary form her impressive and creative skills."

I feel he is right, bless his kind words – I add a touch of creative flair and imagination and joy to everything I do, be it writing or gardening or baking or housesitting. This applies to both my work and play, which are quite yin-and-yang intertwined. I like to think my HAPPY book here is me bringing my light out from under the bushel – not just for family and friends, but for the whole world. I'm sure Ron will be happy about that, too.

And I mentioned housesitting! Something that for me truly embodied 'doing something that brings you joy' as a means to creating your happiness. Well, it was never my intention to become a housesitter; I 'fell into it' by chance, and how glad I am that I did. One time as a favour for a friend, I was 'babysitting' her farm property and her gorgeous Dalmatian dog, Judy. For my 'excellent efforts' my friend rewarded me afterwards with a little stay at her holiday unit in the beautiful Queensland beachside town of Noosa. And so the word spread – "Marie minds houses!" – as a few friends commented to their friends, and those friends passed it on, and so on and so forth… And then VOILÀ, I became a housesitter, all over the place!

I became the Yes Lady whenever I was asked to housesit, and before I knew it I found myself booked YEARS in advance, and I had to 'find time' for my own friends, and daily and social catch-ups. Unexpectedly, my work became my play and my play became my work, equating to a magical 30-odd years of doing this. While I have moments now that I miss it, I was so blessed for so long, and I choose to be happy about it. I met many wonderful people, visited many wonderful places, and minded so many darling pets, that it has all added to my wholehearted happiness, at the time and in my memories now.

One of the great additional pleasures of housesitting was free time – free time to write, read, and send letters, and personal time away from the stresses of general life. It's interesting the feeling you get when you are not rushed, or not in the space of immediate responsibility. Most cats, dogs, birds, unusual pets (even an owl!), plus gardens, antiques and the actual house of the housesit itself, didn't 'need me' immediately or all the time. So where they didn't need my 24/7 attention, my body and my mind became at peace and at full rest. I could get out my own pen and paper, and together with my words and experiences I could let my pen get away into imaginative realms. I wrote much of the content of **Marie's Work and Play** while housesitting and dreaming and remembering. My love for unicorns was the catalyst to a story about 'Sparkles', a naughty unicorn who gave children rides across the solar system. My memories of a bear called Athabaska from my Canadian travel adventures years prior produced a story about a gentle bear doctor character called Doctor Hug-me. And I wrote down my experiences and memories of my housesitting itself, especially about my little furred or feathered friends from the houses…

On the following page is one of my early housesitting tales, a version of which previously appeared in my **Marie's Work and Play** booklet – it made me happy to remember and write it and I hope it makes you happy to read it. More recently I have included many more of my housesitting memories and pet tales in my chapter in Volume 2 of **The New Rules of Wellness** (please see page 87 for where to buy a copy of that book). I loved all of my housesitting and I loved all of my little animal friends, and I'm sure they loved me too. If I miss them now, I can re-read my tales, or I just simply sit and remember them. And then my cup is full. I am happy. I choose to be happy.

Prince on Wheels

Many years ago I often housesat at a Melbourne suburban motel while the owners took regular breaks. Along with the motel came Prince, a dear little dachshund dog, and Ginger, a distinguished orange cat. They were the best of canine and feline friends – they had grown up together and were no trouble to each other or to me at all.

At mealtimes Prince had been trained to wait until Ginger had eaten first, before he was to dine. Prince was a royal gentleman and would sit so patiently.

Because dachshunds are prone to back weakness as they age, Prince's spine had eventually grown too old for his legs. His continuing need for mobility resulted in the invention of a skateboard/harness combination that he wore so that he could still get around – and he never skipped a beat!

The only thing that actually changed was that instead of sitting regally at meals, Prince would gently rock back and forth on his skateboard as he waited for Ginger to finish his food. So Prince became a rocking and rolling royal boy and did very well – maybe getting only a *little* more impatient with his dinner companion as the years clicked by!

4. One More Note of Happiness.

My earliest memory is from when I was three years old. I was sitting on the bonnet of the Chevrolet truck that my father had built. The number plate was registered in the Australian state of Victoria, as '191-420'. Today as I sit here and write, I also reflect on my amazing life and all my work, play, experiences and tiny moments that are so important to me, each and every one of them. This little memory is the first of them.

My father was born in Scotland in May 1901. He came to Australia for a better life. He met Mother at a train station café up in country Victoria where she was working, and he made sure he went and ate there regularly so he could see her. I was born in December 1934, the first of two children from my parents' marriage. We lived in the country and I grew up in the Australian bush.

Dad worked so hard in the Mallee, where he ran Clydesdale draft horses. What a man he was! He grew, he built and he fathered so well, and as a grandfather he would let the kids paint his fingernails with polish, and yell from the 'sit-outery' (the outhouse toilet) that he was okay.

Dad passed away in 1988. I miss him every day of my life. I realise I have outlived my father's age and my mother's too, and I feel blessed for every minute I had with them, and for every minute I have with my family and my grandchildren. So very many wonderful memories.

When I look at the photo of myself on Dad's truck, it feels like it was yesterday. I 'see' and I 'feel' how simple life can be – as we age, we complicate it all. I'm sitting on the bonnet of the truck and I can feel the warmed metal. The wind blows in my hair and over my feet, and the gum trees around me whisper their natural sounds as their leaves rub together. I feel that happiness was a light and lovely part of life just as much for my three-year-old self then as it is for my 89-year-old self now.

I am so glad that I was taught at a young age to always live with inner happiness, and to appreciate the little things. I have done so over my long and remarkable life, and I still do.

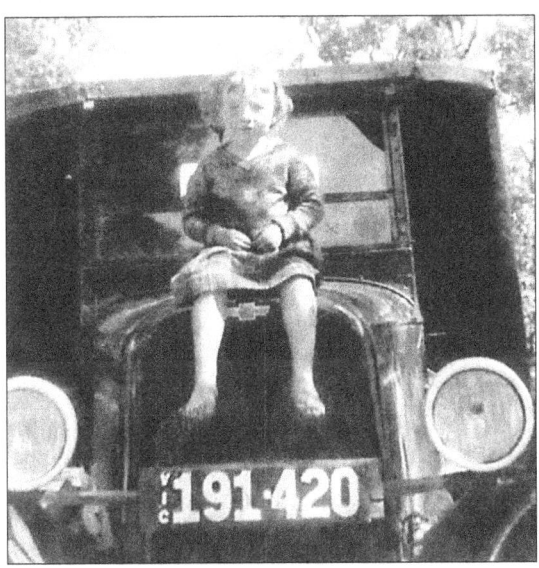

Quick Finder – Recipes Index

The 14 recipes I have included in this book appear in Chapter 2 under the ABCs for happiness, although I admit to being a little creative with their naming and the letters to which they have been assigned!

To make sure that my readers can easily and happily locate just each particular recipe itself, below is a plainly named, alphabetical index of where every full recipe in this book can be found.

Happy cooking, happy baking, and happy EATING!

Apple and rhubarb crumble	page 11
Banana bread	page 14
Coconut loaf cake	page 61
Crêpes Suzette	page 22
Haricot bean hummus	page 27
Hummingbird cake	page 39
Italian seasoning	page 28
Lemon butter syrup cake	page 33
Tomato and onion pie	page 50
Tomato relish	page 45
Treacle tart	page 59
Vanilla muffins	page 54
Walnut and feta hot-roasted beetroot	page 56
Zucchini soup	page 64

Contributions to Other Publications

Marie Elson as author of a chapter or section

SPRUIK IT!: Cultivating the Willingness to Back Yourself to Your Success. Barnes and Noble, 2022. LivingLovingly Press. USA.
  Currently available from:
  - Barnes & Noble

The New Rules of Wellness: Transformational Stories from Health Experts Who Lead from the Heart. Volume 2. House of Wellness Publishing, 2024. Australia.
  Currently available (as is Volume 1!) from:
  - Amazon
  - Barnes & Noble

Marie Elson as a co-author

My Mind is Ever New. Puzzle book and metaphysical vibes. House of Wellness Publishing, 2025 release. Australia.

Praise for 'I Choose To Be Happy'

"Happiness does come from within – I wholeheartedly agree! Some great little tips here that I had never thought of before!" - Angel H, Australia.

"I love a book of transformation! So many nuggets of gold here, and loving the traditional recipes. Highly recommended." - April D, USA.

"This book has given me permission for freedom." - Hannah Mann, Australia.

"Courage is what I've taken from this great little book." - Dani M-S, Canada.

"A cosy mix of motivational and practical advice, sweet little anecdotes, and mouth-watering recipes. Wonderful!" - R Adams, Australia.

"I love the compiled wisdom and understanding within this publication. A very valuable insight." - JW, Australia.

"I really like the little by-stories. Presented wonderfully, and very engaging." - Tina, UK.

"My mother is such an inspiration, and a Force of Happiness! Thank you for being you, Mum!" - Dr. Dee Hacking, Australia.

Author's Message and Thanks

Thank you for checking out my book – I hope you enjoyed my thoughts on happiness. If something in this book might help you to nurture your own happiness, then that also adds to mine!

A huge thank you to Dr. Dee Hacking for editorial assistance, and for her loving and endless support. Thank you to A. W. D. McIntosh for editorial assistance, and for the cover photo of Rosebud Beach.

With love to all my family and friends, whose happiness always enhances my own.

This book is dedicated to my chief happiness and the loves of my life – my incredible daughter, Dr. Dee Hacking, and my two wonderful grandchildren, Dani and Ethan.

Socials:
I don't have my own social media, but please feel free to leave a message for me via Dr. Dee's Facebook page at:
https://www.facebook.com/nereda.hacking

In loving memory of Mother and Dad

Marie McIntosh & Robert McIntosh

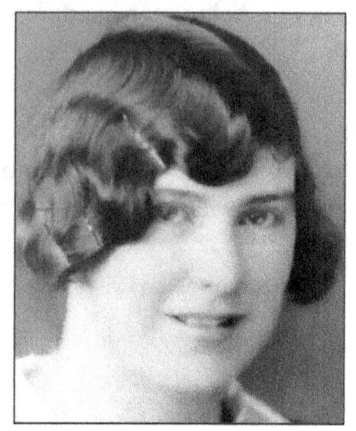
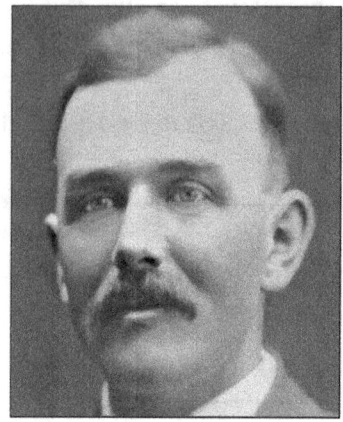

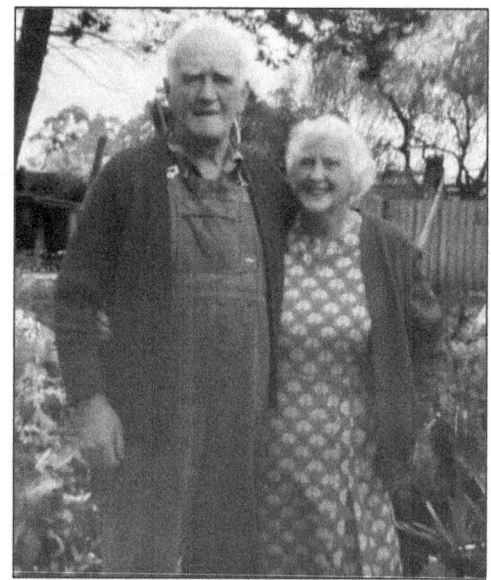

Publisher's Message (Get in Touch!)

House of Wellness Publishing is a boutique publisher created and run by Dr. Dee Hacking. Its purpose is spreading true tales of health, wellness and inspiration, along with stories of fiction (including novels and short story collections), and so much MORE!

Dr. Dee originally hails from Melbourne, Australia, but for many years has made her home in the Queensland coastal town of Mackay, where she runs her own highly regarded health clinic (*Bay Massage & Homeopathy Allied Health Clinic - Dr. Dee*) as well as her publishing business.

Dr. Dee is delighted to be making her mother Marie's dream come true by publishing **I Choose To Be Happy**.

- If it is also your dream to be a published author, perhaps you have something you would like to talk about with Dr. Dee? She would love to hear from you via her socials below. Even if you don't think you have something to say **about** wellness, there's a very broad spectrum of subjects and stories that could help **promote** wellness in our readers, so let's have a chat!

House of Wellness Publishing is the originator of the international bestselling **The New Rules of Wellness** (NROW) series. You can find the published NROW volumes on Amazon. *Author submissions for chapters in our upcoming NROW volumes are currently open (2024-2025)* – please contact us via the **email** below to discuss.

Email: houseofwellnesspublishing@gmail.com
Facebook: https://www.facebook.com/nereda.hacking
LinkedIn: Dr. Dee Hacking

www.ingramcontent.com/pod-product-compliance
Lightning Source LLC
Chambersburg PA
CBHW072017290426
44109CB00018B/2268